Peri-Implant Soft Tissue Management

Mohamed Hassan
Editor

Peri-Implant Soft Tissue Management

A Clinical Guide

Springer

Editor
Mohamed Hassan
Oral Medicine, Infection & Immunity
Harvard Dental School
Boston, MA, USA

ISBN 978-3-031-45515-5 ISBN 978-3-031-45516-2 (eBook)
https://doi.org/10.1007/978-3-031-45516-2

This Springer imprint is published by the registered company Springer Nature Switzerland AG
The registered company address is: Gewerbestrasse 11, 6330 Cham, Switzerland

Paper in this product is recyclable

Contents

1 Introduction: Dental Implants and Soft Tissues: Roles and Challenges

Mohamed Hassan

Dental implants have become a widely accepted modality for replacing missing teeth to fulfill both the functional, aesthetic, and other needs of patients. Adequate supporting structures (bone and soft tissues) are essential to achieving high implant success rates. While adequate quantity and quality of bone play a major role in the short and long-term implant support, proper soft tissue management contributes to both functional and aesthetic outcomes.

This book highlights different modalities and techniques for handling soft tissues from the surgical phase and through and beyond the restorative phase. The aim of the book is to provide dentists who are involved in dental implants with an overview of how to deal with challenges they may face regarding soft tissues as related to supporting the placement of implants.

1.1 Multi-Stakeholder and Multifactor Approaches to Supporting the Management of Soft Tissues

Tooth loss can pose a challenge to patients and negatively affect many aspects of their lives, including social, physical, and mental health. Due to the importance of the presence of teeth to facilitate chewing food, phonetics, and aesthetics, edentulism may negatively impact the quality of life.

Dentists across specialties and other dental professionals (e.g., hygienists, dental assistants) ongoingly need to expand our knowledge base in order to meet patients' priorities and circumstances in manners that fit their lifestyle and maintain an acceptable quality of life throughout the process. Patients expect their dental care

M. Hassan (✉)
Oral Medicine, Infection & Immunity, Harvard School of Dental Medicine, Boston, MA, USA
e-mail: Mohamed_Hassan@hsdm.harvard.edu

M. Hassan (ed.), *Peri-Implant Soft Tissue Management*,
https://doi.org/10.1007/978-3-031-45516-2_1

providers to be able to discuss different treatment options with them and help them make choices that best fit their needs.

For dentists to effectively meet patients' needs, they should be familiar with different methods of tooth replacement and the advantages and limitations of each option as pertaining to the circumstances of each patient. Currently, dental implants are considered the option that most patients and dental health care providers consider the closest match to natural dentitions.

If patients opt to have implants replace their missing teeth, it becomes essential to establish a dialogue to discuss how to implement logistical steps to promote success. Patients and members of the dental team need to be familiar with all the treatment steps involved in order to avoid misunderstandings, lack of coordination, and other unsatisfactory outcomes for all parties. Successful outcomes are a shared responsibility between patients and their dental care team.

Promoting a high success rate of implants is a multifactorial process. Some factors are related to the patient's medical, dental, anatomical, and functional conditions. Other factors are related to the ability of the dental team to prepare and deal with clinical findings during different stages of implant placement. One of the most important factors that significantly affects the success rate of dental implants is the presence of adequate and healthy hard and soft tissues. This textbook focuses on the soft tissues around dental implants and varied techniques of dealing with their lack of quantity or quality. Bringing together medical doctors and dentists, we provide a holistic perspective on how all members of the dental team can collaborate across the surgical, restorative, and even maintenance phases to support positive outcomes and increase the success rate of dental implants.

1.2 Overview of Chapters

The chapters outline ways to deal with multiple aspects of soft tissue deficiencies to ensure the proper quantity and quality surrounding dental implants. In addition to helping correct existing problems, the chapters address ways to maintain healthy conditions once achieved in order to prevent potential future deformities. Achieving and maintaining healthy soft tissues will help increase the implant success rate with increased longevity.

In particular, Chap. 2 (Hassan, A) describes that in order to make a sound and clear treatment plan, practitioners need to familiarize themselves with the histology and anatomy of different types of oral soft tissues. Without adequate and correct anatomical and histological knowledge, clinicians may face challenges in how to diagnose and manage the clinical situation based on a patient's needs and circumstances.

The overview of histology and anatomy provides the foundation for Chap. 3 (Jeong), which focuses on the role of soft tissues in long-term success of dental implants. Long-term implant success depends on the unique characteristics of each type of soft tissue.

To achieve long-term success, dentists need to manage short-term challenges, as described in Chap. 4 (Hassan, M.), which describes soft tissue management during different stages of surgical placement of implants. Once dentists determine a deficiency in either the quality and quantity of soft tissues, clinicians usually have multiple chances and phases to augment the quantity and/or improve the quality of existing soft tissues surrounding the site of the implant before, during, and after its placement. Chapter 4 reviews multiple methods and techniques that can be utilized in various stages in case an aspect of supporting soft tissues is not completed at a particular stage. Having a range of methods and opportunities to implement them, including the surgical or even after loading the implants, allows practitioners to choose the most applicable or appropriate method based on clinical evaluation and timing of the procedure.

Once the implant is placed and/or loaded, Chap. 5 (Kim and colleagues) stresses the importance of maintenance to help continue its success. Routine maintenance visits and proper oral hygiene measures are needed to maintain healthy soft tissue around dental implants and promote the longevity of the implant. Maintenance of dental implants includes periodic clinical and radiographic evaluations to facilitate early detection of and dealing with potential failure or negative signs or symptoms. Periodic visits also allow dental care providers to achieve adequate patient compliance and knowledge of home care and oral hygiene instructions with the use of different brushing techniques and hygiene instruments. These nonsurgical measures minimize the need for more invasive surgical techniques.

Despite all the measures taken to ensure healthy and adequate soft tissues, practitioners who are involved in dental implant work may encounter soft tissue pathology, which may affect the longevity and success of the implants. Chapter 6 (Alaskar) offers an overview of the most common pathologic lesions and proper surgical and nonsurgical measures to manage them. In cases of soft tissue pathology, treatment planning should be determined through consultations between clinicians (e.g., general dentists, pathologists, and implantologists).

Implants may show signs and present symptoms of failure and or adverse outcomes and different stages during the complete treatment journey. While the surgical team is mainly responsible for the first stage of surgical preparation of implant placement, the restorative team will complement the surgical phase by fabricating and inserting a well fitted, functioning, and aesthetically accepted restoration. In order to provide patients with a comprehensively determined treatment plan that is implemented in a coordinated manner, sound communication between different practitioners is essential throughout the stages of implant placement and its restoration. Assuming the surgical phase is completed, Chap. 7 (Khamis) reviews the prosthetic role in peri-implant during the treatment planning phase. In particular, the chapter outlines relevant theory or rationale and the corresponding methods of prosthetic contribution to peri-implant soft tissue management. The chapter reviews a range of factors that need to be taken into consideration in relation to patient selection, aesthetic treatment planning and implant positioning, and emergence profile while achieving a properly contoured final restoration.

Adequate knowledge is necessary to help make an educated decision to select between all the available types of restoration. Chapter 8 (Khamis) presents the steps involved in the selection between various prosthetic designs and their effects on peri-implant soft tissues, whether it is screw or cement-retained restoration.

Finally, once the implant has been restored, Chap. 9 (Hassan, M) emphasizes the effects of occlusion on the long-term success and health of dental implants. Inadequate consideration of the effects of occlusion may lead to implant failure in the long term as it may contribute to excessive bone loss and soft tissue inadequacy. After reviewing different types of occlusion, the chapter focuses on traumatic occlusion as a common factor to show its negative effects on implants and their surrounding hard and soft tissues.

This volume confirms how implant success requires multifactorial management of soft tissues and other relevant factors by knowledgeable members of the dental team who collaborate effectively with one another and communicate clearly with the patient to set and work towards reasonable expectations about the case. Without adequate knowledge about the role of each member and coordination between them, the results may be compromised, and the outcomes may be unsatisfactory to all dental providers and patients. The high cost to manage and correct undesirable outcomes or to meet the patient's demands can often be avoided if the patient's expectations are adjusted to reflect the current situation.

Accordingly, this volume highlights different modalities and techniques for handling soft tissues from the surgical phase and through and beyond the restorative phase in order to provide dentists with an overview of how to deal with challenges regarding soft tissues as related to supporting the placement of implants.

Histology and Anatomy of Different Types of Oral Mucosa

2

Abdelghany Hassan Abdelghany

2.1 Anatomy of the Oral Mucosa

The human oral cavity is lined by a mucous membrane (the oral mucosa) that seems to be more complicated than it first appears. The oral mucosa is made up of a stratified squamous epithelium, which may or may not be keratinized. It varies from site to site within the oral cavity, but everywhere the epithelium is protective stratified squamous [1, 2] (Fig. 2.1).

The oral cavity has sometimes been described as a mirror that reflects the health of the individual [3]. Changes indicative of disease are seen as alterations in the oral mucosa lining the mouth, which can reveal systemic conditions, such as diabetes or vitamin deficiency, or the local effects of chronic tobacco or alcohol use [4].

Oral mucosa can be divided into three main categories based on function and histology: masticatory, lining, and specialized mucosa.

1. ***Masticatory mucosa***, keratinized stratified squamous epithelium, found on the dorsum of the tongue, hard palate, and attached gingiva [6] (Figs. 2.2, 2.3, 2.4).

   The **hard palate** has a partially-keratinized epithelium, much of which is firmly attached by a fibrous submucosa to underlying bone. This epithelium is partially keratinized on gums and hard palate [6] (Figs. 2.1, 2.4).

A. H. Abdelghany (✉)
Department of Anatomy and Embryology, Faculty of Medicine, Alexandria University, Alexandria, Egypt

Faculty of Medicine, Arab Academy for Science, Technology and Maritime Transport, Alamein, Egypt

Faculty of Medicine, Alexandria National University, Alexandria, Egypt

Anatomy Lead of Manchester Program, Faculty of Medicine, Alexandria University, Alexandria, Egypt
e-mail: abdulghani.abdulghani@alexmed.edu.eg

M. Hassan (ed.), *Peri-Implant Soft Tissue Management*,
https://doi.org/10.1007/978-3-031-45516-2_2

Fig. 2.1 Mouth cavity

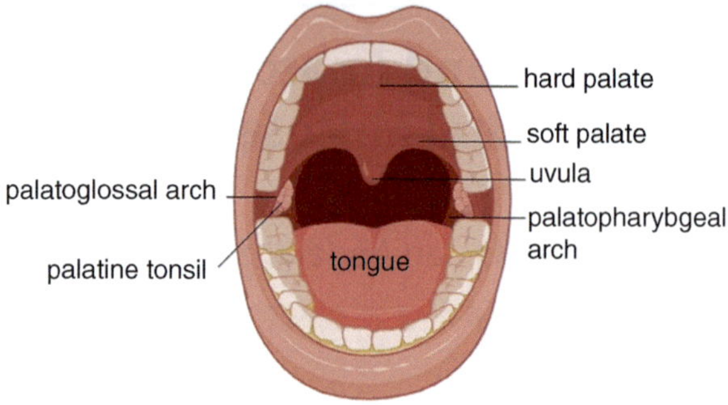

Fig. 2.2 Mouth cavity [5]

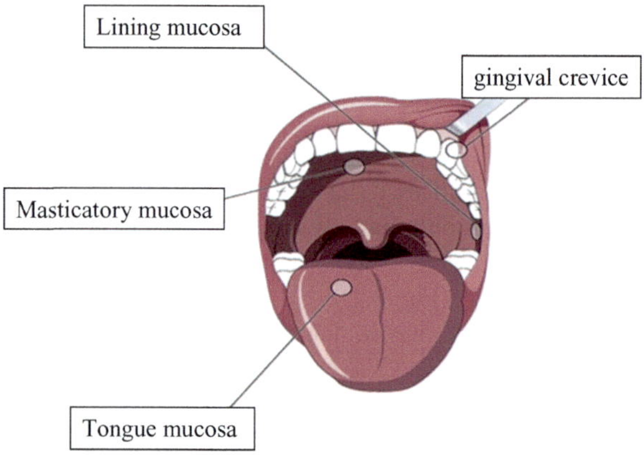

Fig. 2.3 Lingual mucosa

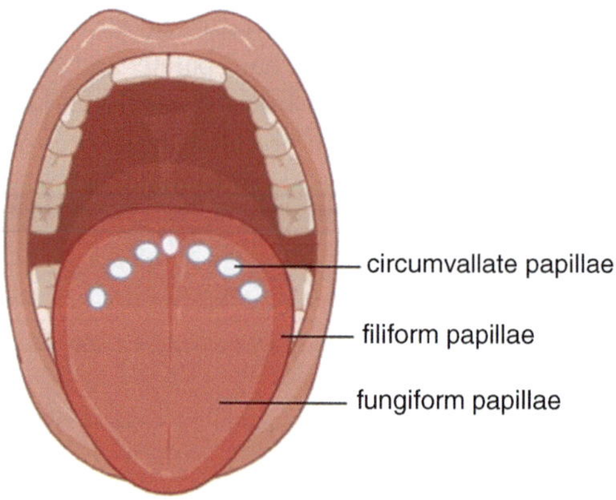

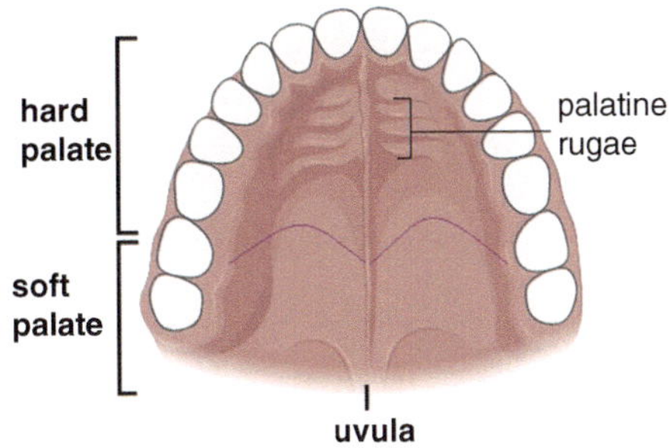

Fig. 2.4 Masticatory mucosa

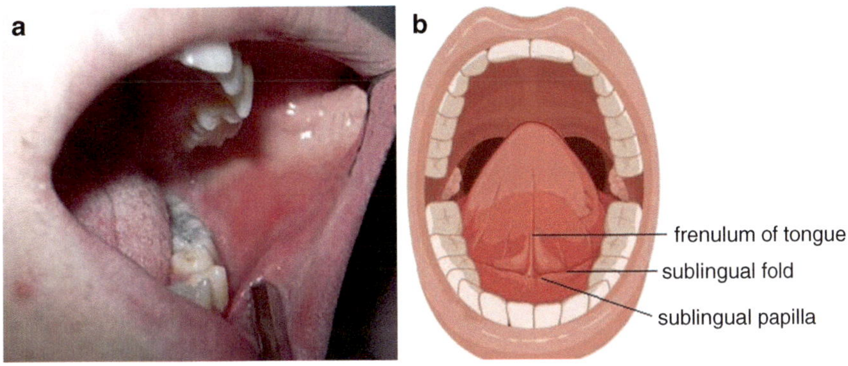

Fig. 2.5 Buccal mucosa on the cheek (**a**) and floor of the mouth (**b**) [8]

2. ***Lining mucosa***, nonkeratinized stratified squamous epithelium, found almost everywhere else in the oral cavity, including the buccal, labial, and alveolar mucosa [6, 7].
   (a) ***Buccal mucosa*** refers to the inside lining of the cheeks and floor of the mouth [7] (Fig. 2.5).
   (b) ***Labial mucosa*** refers to the inside lining of the lips. It is the moist internal portion of the lip [7] (Fig. 2.6).
   (c) ***Alveolar mucosa*** refers to the covering of the alveolar process of the maxillae and mandible. It is continuous with the mucosa of the cheek, lips, and palate and is loosely attached to the underlying bone [6, 7] (Fig. 2.7).
      - It is easily distinguished by its bright red color due to many blood vessels and its smooth shiny surface [6].
3. ***Specialized mucosa,*** specifically in the regions of the taste buds on lingual papillae on the dorsal surface of the tongue that contains nerve endings for general sensory reception and taste perception [7] (Figs. 2.3, 2.8).

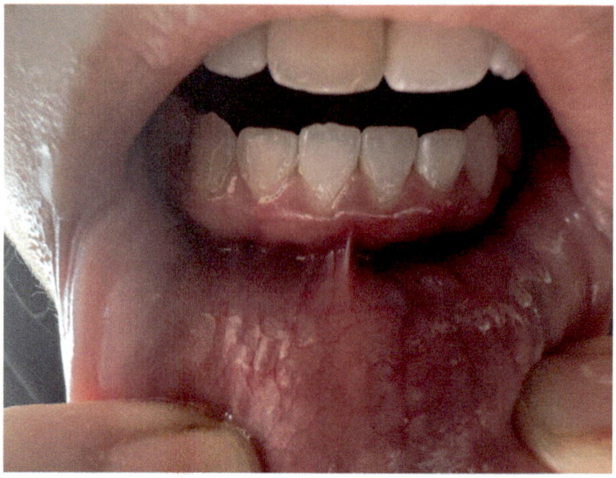

Fig. 2.6 Labial mucosa [9]

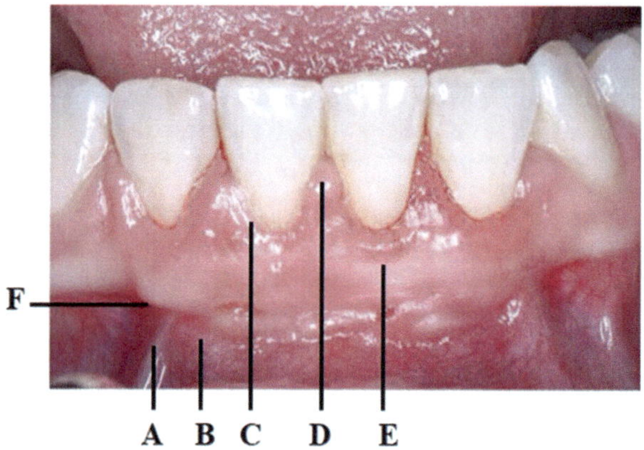

Fig. 2.7 Alveolar mucosa [9]. (**a**) Attached gingiva. (**b**) Alveolar mucosa. (**c**) Interdental papilla. (**d**) Free gingiva. (**e**) Labial frenulum. (**f**) Mucogingival junction

A. Attached gingiva.
B. Alveolar mucosa.
C. Interdental papilla.
D. Free gingiva.
E. Labial frenulum.
F. Mucogingival junction.

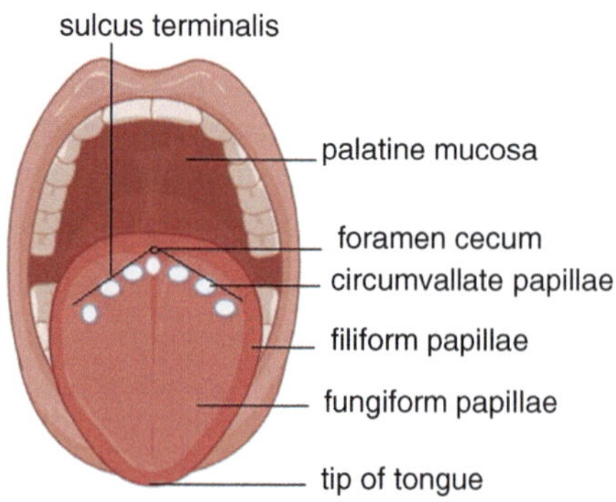

Fig. 2.8 Specialized mucosa

2.2 Histology of the Oral Mucosa

The human buccal mucosa is made up of various layers and levels. It contains four independent layers and an underlying connective tissue layer, the lamina propria. The surface is kept moist with mucus produced by the major and numerous minor salivary glands. The oral mucosa is well supplied with nerve endings and, on the dorsal surface of the tongue, special sensory endings for taste [1].

2.2.1 Layers of the Oral Mucosa

2.2.1.1 Stratum Basale

The stratum basale (also called the stratum germinativum) is the deepest of the layers of the buccal mucosa. The stratum basale is formed of a continuous layer, usually only one cell thick, of short cuboidal to columnar stem cells. The basement membrane of the cells of this layer is represented by intertwining collagen fibers that help bind these cells to the deeper layers.

The cells of the stratum basale, basal keratinocytes, are considered the stem cells of the buccal mucosa. The primary function of these keratinocytes is to divide by going through successive mitotic divisions, generating new cells that migrate superficially to the next superficial mucosal layer, stratum spinosum, in the process of renewal of the mucosal cells.

The newly formed cells will undergo a progressive maturation called keratinization as they migrate to the surface of the mucosa [1] (Fig. 2.9).

2.2.1.2 Stratum Spinosum

The stratum spinosum (or spinous layer or prickle cell layer) is the layer of buccal mucosa found superficial to the stratum basale and deeper to the stratum granulosum [1, 3]. As the name implies, this layer is spiny in appearance due to the presence of dcsmosomcs, which arc protruding ccll spiky microfilamcnt projections that join the cells in close contact (Figs. 2.9, 2.10).

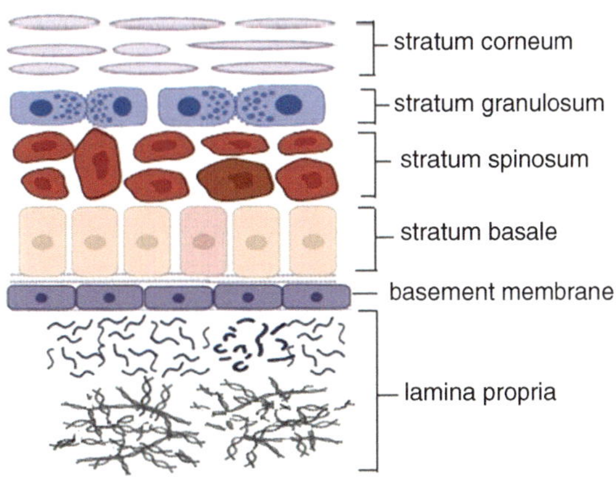

Fig. 2.9 Schematic illustration of the layers found in the keratinized oral mucosa

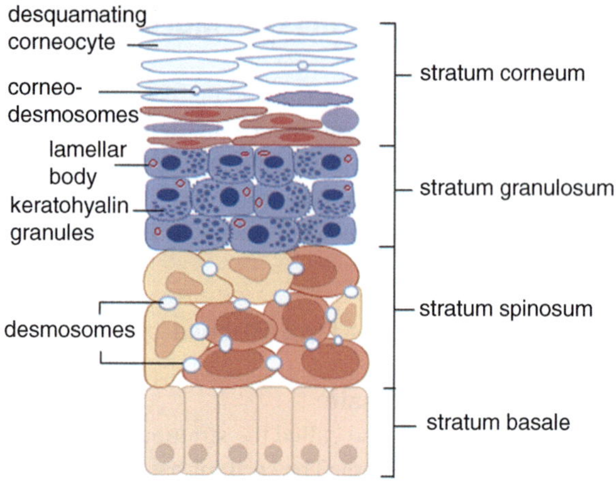

Fig. 2.10 Layers of the oral mucosa

The stratum spinosum is composed of 8 to 10 layers of polyhedral keratinocytes which are formed as a result of successive cell division in the stratum basale. These cells are active in synthesizing fibrillar proteins, known as cytokeratin, which builds up within the cells, aggregating together and forming prominent bundles of keratin microfilaments that go on to form the desmosomes, which allow for strong connections to form between the adjacent keratinocytes. These desmosomes interlock with each other and strengthen the bond between the cells. Therefore, the process of keratinization starts in the stratum spinosum [4, 9].

These spine-like structures are believed to serve as the underlying structural reinforcements that provide strength, elasticity, and flexibility to the layers of the oral mucosa and to better withstand the effects of friction and abrasion. Moreover, the keratinocytes in the stratum spinosum release a water-repelling glycolipid, rendering the mucosa relatively waterproof. As new keratinocytes are produced in the stratum basale, the keratinocytes of the stratum spinosum are pushed upward to the stratum granulosum [4, 9].

2.2.1.3 Stratum Granulosum

It is considered a transitional layer sandwiched between the metabolically active layers beneath, stratum basale and stratum spinosum, and the non-viable layer, stratum corneum (containing dead cells) above.

It is a thin layer of 3 to 5 cell layers thick. When the keratinocytes are pushed from the stratum spinosum, they become flatter, their cell membranes thicken, and they generate large amounts of the protein keratin, which is fibrous. It is chiefly involved in providing waterproofing function. It also contributes to the keratinization process of the mucosa [4, 9].

It is referred to as the granular layer, as the cells contain irregularly shaped granules. There are two types of granules formed in this layer: the basophilic keratohyalin and the lamellar granules formed by the lamellar bodies (Figs. 2.9, 2.10).

The basophilic keratohyalin granules contain keratohyalin protein, which is rich in histidine and cysteine. Therefore, the cells are able to generate large amounts of the fibrous protein, keratin. In this way, they seem to be deeply involved in keratinization (formation of keratin) by binding the keratin microfilaments together so that the bundles of keratin become more prominent. Thus, the process of keratinization actually begins in this layer [4, 6].

Also, keratohyalin granules promote dehydration of the cells so that as the cells move toward the stratum granulosum, their nuclei begin to show certain changes, they get flattened with dense masses of nuclear chromatin and early signs of breaking up of the nuclear membrane. It is thought that the lysosomal membranes rupture with the release of lysosomal enzymes, which are responsible for the breakdown of the cells and eventually cause cell death [7, 9, 10].

On the other hand, the lamellar granules secrete a lipid-rich substance that accumulates in the extracellular space between the cells of the stratum granulosum and coats their membranes making them thicker. This lipid-rich material ensures that the cells are firmly connected together and also forms a waterproof barrier. In other words, the lipids by acting as water sealant make the layer waterproof, and moreover, also reduce its permeability and prevent water and water-soluble substances from passing through and entering the lower layers. Penetration of any foreign material or microbes is also not possible [11, 12] (Figs. 2.9, 2.10).

At the transition between this layer and the stratum corneum, the nuclei and other cell organelles disintegrate and the cells die, leaving dark cytoplasmic material and densely packed keratin filaments within the cell membranes. So, when these nonviable cells reach the above layer (stratum corneum), they turn dead and fully packed with keratin and now they are called corneocytes [9].

2.3 Stratum Corneum

The stratum corneum is the most superficial and exposed layer of the oral mucosa. The increased keratinization (also called cornification) of the cells in this layer gives it its name. There are usually 15–30 layers of cells in the stratum corneum. This dry, dead layer helps prevent the penetration of microbes and the dehydration of underlying tissues and provides mechanical protection against abrasion for the more delicate, underlying layers. Moreover, it is the keratin that makes the mucosa flexible and strong. Cells in this layer are shed periodically and are replaced by cells pushed up from the stratum granulosum [9] (Figs. 2.9, 2.10).

2.3.1 Movement of Keratinocytes from the Stratum Basale to the Superficial Layers

As new cells are produced in the stratum basale, the keratinocytes of the stratum spinosum are constantly being pushed toward the next layer, the stratum granulosum, where the keratinocytes secrete keratin and lipids that serve as the skin's waterproof barrier. Then, the cells begin to lose their nuclei and organelles and become dead in the outermost layer, the stratum corneum. It takes approximately 14 days for a cell to migrate from the stratum basale to the stratum corneum and further 2 weeks for the cells to cross the stratum corneum to the surface, where they finally are shed. Injury and inflammation increase the rate of proliferation and maturation [9].

2.4 N.B.

Most of the oral mucosa consists of parakeratinized epithelium, which contains nucleated keratinocytes. Parakeratinized epithelium is a term usually used for partially keratinized epithelium that doesn't have several layers of dead cells at the surface, as may be found in the oral cavity.

Parakeratinized epithelium is similar to keratinized epithelium, except that in parakeratinized epithelium, cell nuclei are present in the stratum corneum. An example is the masticatory mucosa located on the hard palate and gingiva [11–13].

2.4.1 The Lamina Propria

It is a layer of fibrous connective tissue that consists of a network of collagen fibers (type I and III). Fibroblasts represent the main cells of the lamina propria, and they are responsible for the production of fibers as well as the extracellular matrix. Other cells, such as lymphocytes, plasma cells, and mast cells, are also present [10, 13] (Fig. 2.11).

The lamina propria helps provide support and nutrition to the epithelium, as well as a means to bind to the underlying tissue [13].

The lamina propria has two layers: papillary and dense.

(a) ***The papillary layer*** is the superficial layer. It consists of connective tissue papillae containing loose areolar connective tissue, along with blood vessels and nerves [12, 13].
(b) ***The dense layer*** is the deeper layer of the lamina propria. It consists of dense connective tissue with a large amount of fibers [13] (Fig. 2.11).

A submucosa may or may not be present deep to the dense layer of the lamina propria, depending on the region of the oral cavity, and it overlies the bones. If present, the submucosa usually contains loose areolar connective tissue with blood vessels and nerves and may also contain adipose tissue or minor salivary glands [10] (Fig. 2.11).

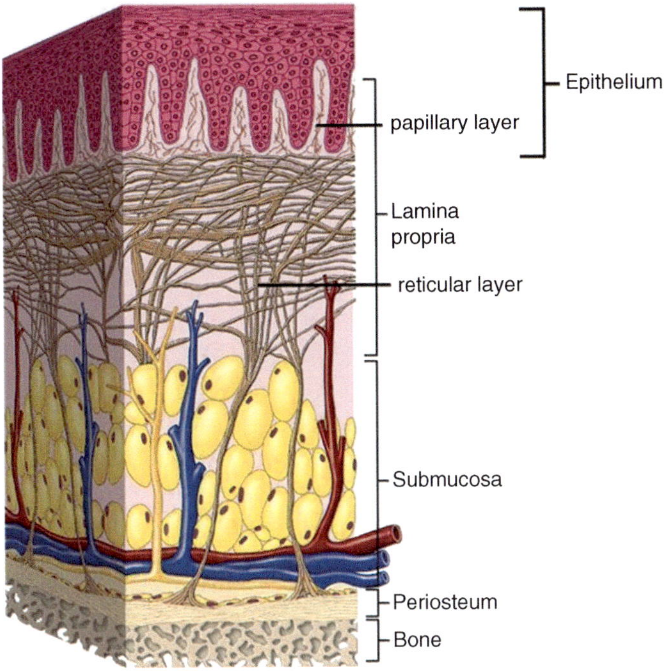

Fig. 2.11 Lamina propria and submucous layer of the oral mucosa [14]

References

1. Nancy A. Structure of the oral tissue. In: Ten cate's oral histology, development, structure and function. 8th ed. Elsevier; 2013. p. 280.
2. Drake RL, Vogl AW, Mitchell AWM, Tibbitts RM, Richardson PE. Head and neck. In: Gray's atlas of anatomy. Chirchill Livingstone, International ed; 2008. p. 428–538.
3. Rosengard HC, Messadi DV, Mirowski GW. Oral manifestations of systemic diseases at eMedicine. 2018.
4. Squier CA, Kremer MJ. Biology of oral mucosa and esophagus. J Natl Cancer Inst Monogr. 2001;29:7 15.
5. Proksch E, Brasch J. Tissue specific immunity at the oral mucosal barrier. Trends Immunol. 2018;39(4):276–87.
6. Chandra S, Chandra S, Chandra M, Chandra G, Chandra N. Textbook of dental and oral histology and embryology with MCQs. 2nd ed. New Delhi: Jaypee Brothers; 2010. p. 180.
7. Fehrenbach M, Popowics T. Illustrated dental embryology, histology, and anatomy. 4th ed. St. Louis, MI: Elsevier; 2015. p. 106.
8. Kal BI, Evcin O, Dundar N, Tezel H, Unal I. An unusual case of immediate hypersensitivity reaction associated with an amalgam restoration. Br Dent J. 2008;205(10):547–50.
9. Berkovitz BK, Holland GH, Moxham BJ. Oral anatomy, histology and embryology. 3rd ed. Mosby; 2002. p. 220–48.

10. Young B, Lowe JS, Stevens A, Heath JW. Wheater's functional histology: a text and colour atlas. 5th ed. Amsterdam: Elsevier; 2007. p. 251–62.
11. Presland RB, Dale BA. Epithelial structural proteins of the skin and oral cavity: function in health and disease. Rev Oral Biol Med. 2000;11(4):383.
12. Presland RB, Jurevic RJ. Making sense of the epithelial barrier: what molecular biology and genetics tell us about the functions of oral mucosal and epidermal tissues. J Dent Educ. 2002;66(4):564.
13. Junqueira LCU, Carneiro J. Basic histology text & atlas. Lang Des. 10th ed; 2003. p. 187.
14. Sapna K, Renuka D, Gholve S. Challenges face by pharmaceutical industry for the development of oral film dosages form. Int J Pharm Pharm Res. 2017;10(1):1.

The Role and Importance of Soft Tissues for Long-Term Success of Dental Implants

3

Y. Natalie Jeong

The demand for dental implants continues to grow because more providers and patients are viewing dental implants as a predictable therapeutic treatment option. With more patients receiving dental implant treatments, treating clinicians are observing more complications and adverse events as well [1–3]. Therefore, the long-term efficacy of dental implants must be carefully assessed. Criteria such as marginal bone level, patient comfort level, and sulcus depth have been used to define the long-term success of implant therapy [1, 2].

Although osseointegration has traditionally been considered the most important factor in maintaining implant stability, the roles of transmucosal healing and health around the implant are also being considered as determining factors that influence long-term implant success [3, 4]. Peri-implant mucosa that forms during the wound healing process following implant placement is the corresponding term for biological width around natural teeth [5, 6]. The basic function of the peri-implant mucosa is to protect the underlying bone that supports the implant [7]. The average peri-implant mucosal dimension is 3 mm, which is 1 mm longer than the biologic width of natural teeth [8]. Although it has been controversial for many years, the preponderance of evidence suggests that a minimum dimension of peri-implant mucosa is crucial in maintaining long-term implant health. Invasion of the peri-implant mucosa results in tissue inflammation and potential bone loss [8–11], and the breakdown and loss of peri-implant tissue can compromise the long-term success and survival of the implant [7].

The soft tissue attachment apparatus around dental implants is significantly different from that of natural teeth [12, 13]. In natural teeth, the root of the tooth is covered by a root cementum from which collagen fibers run perpendicular to the long axis of

Y. N. Jeong (✉)
Department of Periodontology, Tufts University School of Dental Medicine, Boston, MA, USA
e-mail: natalie.jeong@tufts.edu

M. Hassan (ed.), *Peri-Implant Soft Tissue Management*,
https://doi.org/10.1007/978-3-031-45516-2_3

the tooth and attach to the surrounding hard and soft tissues. An implant has no cementum, and the collagen fibers are oriented parallel to the long axis of the implant without direct anchorage [12–14]. Therefore, the peri-implant soft tissues are more fragile during the inflammatory process [15, 16]. Clinical soft-tissue parameters such as tissue phenotype, amount of keratinized mucosa, and tissue thickness have been considered important factors that influence long-term implant success [17–20]. According to a study that examined peri-implant mucosal dimension using bone sounding around the implants, a peri-implant mucosal dimension at the facial aspect of less than 3 mm was associated with a thin biotype. A thick biotype was observed when there was a peri-implant mucosal dimension of more than 4 mm at the facial aspect. Implant restoration may be prone to papilla loss when the distance from the tip of the papilla to the bone of the adjacent tooth is greater than 4 mm in a thin biotype [5].

To maintain long-term stable implant health, a minimum peri-implant dimension is necessary. Violation of peri-implant mucosa causes peri-implant tissue inflammation and marginal bone loss, and angular defects may develop [9–12].

3.1 Peri-Implant Phenotype

The peri-implant phenotype is defined as "the morphologic and dimensional features characterizing the clinical presentation of the tissue that surround and support osseointegrated implants" [21]. The components of the peri-implant phenotype are keratinized mucosa width (KMW), mucosal tissue thickness (MTT), and supracrestal tissue height (STH). The peri-implant bone thickness makes up the osseous component of the peri-implant phenotype [21] (Fig. 3.1). This description applies to

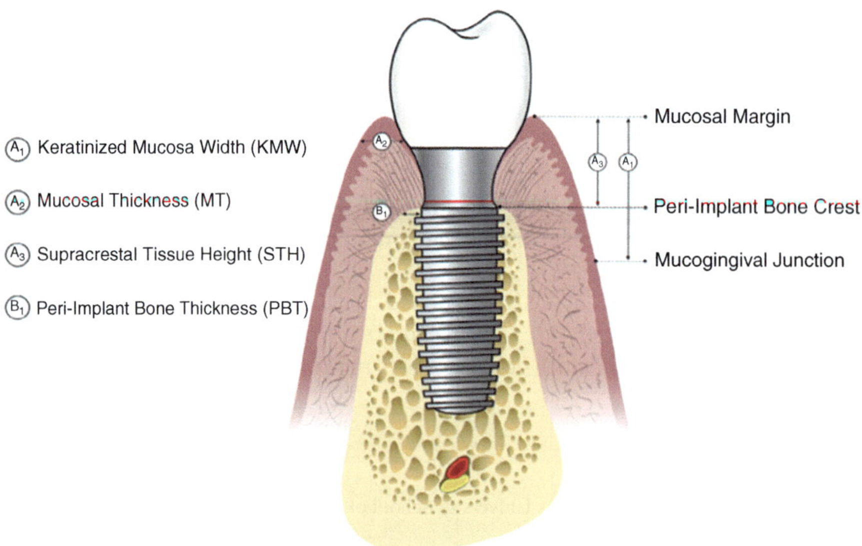

Fig. 3.1 The components of the peri-implant phenotype (adapted from Avila-Ortiz G, Gonzales-Martin O, Couso-Queiruga E, Wang HL [21])

the lingual and facial aspects of the implants. The peri-implant phenotype is site-specific and may change because of external factors [21]. The thick labial peri-implant phenotype is present when there is a thick buccal plate [17]. Furthermore, the peri-implant soft tissue phenotype may be modified with surgical interventions [22]. Therefore, clinicians may consider intervention by means of bone augmentation before or during implant placement when a thin buccal plate is present [17].

3.2 Keratinized Mucosa Width

Keratinized mucosa extends from the margin of the peri-implant mucosa to the oral mucosa [23]. The peri-implant KMW is the most coronal part of the peri-implant soft tissues [21]. The need for adequate width of keratinized mucosa around dental implants has been studied by many researchers and remains somewhat controversial [20, 24–31]. At present, the consensus seems to be that an adequate KMW is associated with low plaque accumulation and improved soft tissue health (Fig. 3.2).

Several studies have shown that in subjects with KMW a greater than 2 mm, the Modified Plaque Index and Modified Gingival Index were higher and the Plaque Index and Gingival Index were lower [20, 27, 31–36]. When probed, implants with a narrow zone of keratinized mucosa tend to bleed more than implants with a wider zone of keratinized mucosa [30, 37, 38]. It has been revealed that implants with a KMW less than 2 mm showed more plaque accumulation and that they were more likely to sustain tissue breakdown, leading to earlier loss of attachment [15, 16, 30, 37, 39]. Pain during home care was reported more frequently by the patients with inadequate KMW at implant sites. This could be caused by mechanical irritation resulting from the mobility of non-keratinized tissue when stimulated by a toothbrush [30]. However, it has also been observed that peri-implant health can be sustained in the presence of inadequate KMW (less than 2 mm) in patients who practice meticulous oral hygiene [28, 29]. Dental implants without adequate KMW, combined with high levels of plaque accumulation, had a greater incidence of peri-implantitis [28, 37–39]. Furthermore, it was found that gingival recession was greater around implants that were not surrounded by adequate KMW compared to the implants with adequate KMW (Fig. 3.3) [31, 32, 36, 38]. Keratinized mucosa

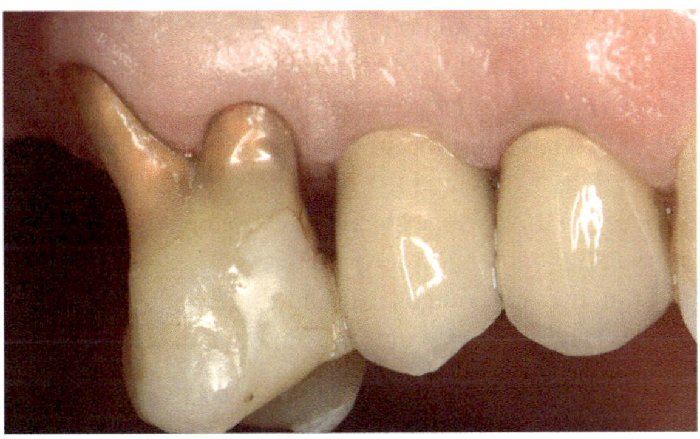

Fig. 3.2 #4 implant with adequate KMW with healthy peri-implant tissue (Photo courtesy of Dr. Andreas Parashis)

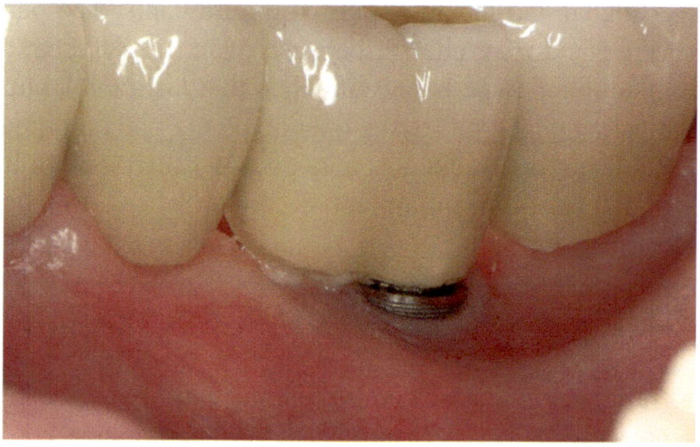

Fig. 3.3 Implant with inadequate KMW and recession (Photo courtesy of Dr. Andreas Parashis)

width can be a key parameter to measure in the timely identification of mucosal recession of dental implants [32, 40]. However, it has been suggested that inadequate KMW may be a consequence of recession, rather than the precipitating factor for worsening of a site [32, 38, 41]. In conclusion, although an adequate KMW may not be a prerequisite for long-term implant health, the presence of adequate KMW may reduce the occurrence of peri-implant tissue inflammation and the breakdown of peri-implant mucosa.

3.3 Mucosal Tissue Thickness

Peri-implant mucosal tissue thickness (MTT), the horizontal dimension of soft tissue, can be measured with a probe at approximately 1.5 mm apical to the soft tissue margin at the base of the probing depth. MTT extends from the external soft tissues to the internal hard surfaces. Peri-implant MTT may or may not be keratinized and does not necessarily correspond to the height of the keratinized tissue. The soft tissue thickness is closely related to the peri-implant phenotype. The dimension may vary from location to location (e.g., facial versus lingual) [21, 42]. The midfacial aspect of the tissue thickness is affected by the implant's shoulder location [43].

The thickness of the peri-implant tissue plays a significant role in the long-term success of implant therapy, as well as functional and esthetic outcomes [21, 44–46]. Implants with thin crestal mucosa tend to have more marginal bone loss than implants with adequate crestal mucosa [47, 48]. Mucosal tissue thickness plays a more significant role in minimizing marginal bone loss with implants that were placed supracrestally compared to implants that were placed at the level of the crest [49, 50]. This could be because of the different locations of the interface between the implant fixture and the implant abutment. Implants with crestal placement have a microgap that is very close to the bone, and marginal bone loss may occur because of potential bacterial microleakage [49].

Implants with mucosal tissue thickness of more than 2 mm, as measured horizontally and perpendicularly from the crest, have low marginal bone loss; therefore, it is suggested to perform autogenous or allogenic tissue grafting to minimize early marginal bone loss [48, 51, 52]. Soft tissue grafting procedures to increase mucosal tissue thickness minimize interproximal marginal bone loss overtime [53]. Additionally, successful outcomes have been achieved when soft tissue augmentation was attempted to enhance esthetics and compensate for an underlying osseous defect. The procedure can be performed before or after the loading of the implants [54, 55]. With the effect of the abutment shade on the peri-implant mucosa, the negative visual consequence was minimized in sites with a minimal mucosal tissue thickness of approximately 2 mm [45, 46].

In conclusion, mucosal tissue thickness must be carefully evaluated by clinicians prior to implant placement because implants placed on the sites with thicker peri-implant soft tissue tend to sustain less marginal bone loss. Furthermore, thin mucosal tissue is a risk factor for esthetic complications because it compromises the appearance of the shade of the abutment [56]. When the thin tissue is noted, the use of soft tissue augmentation with allograft or autogenous graft should be considered to minimize peri-implant marginal bone loss and improve the esthetic outcome. Clinicians should make every effort to achieve and maintain a minimum of 2 mm of mucosal tissue thickness in daily clinical practice.

3.4 Supracrestal Tissue Height

The supracrestal tissue height (STH) is the "vertical dimension of the soft tissue," which runs from the mucosal margin to the bone crest; this is assessed "circumferentially" around an implant, at both proximal sites and buccal and lingual aspects [21]. This characteristic can be measured by transmucosal sounding with a periodontal probe [56]. "Vertical soft tissue thickness on crestal bone" is another term that is used to refer STH [51]. The sulcular epithelium, the junctional epithelium, and the supracrestal connective tissue are engirdled in the peri-implant STH. The supracrestal connective tissue is not directly attached to the implant abutment surface [21]. The dimension of the peri-implant STH is different from its counterpart, the supracrestal tissue attachment of the tooth, in that it is taller by 1 to 1.5 mm in all buccal/lingual and proximal aspects. It is typically greater in interproximal areas [23].

An inadequate STH at the time of implant placement surgery is a predisposing factor for early marginal bone loss [47, 48, 51], regardless of the type of implant (e.g., bone level implant, tissue level implant, or implant with platform switching) [21]. This is probably due to the physiologic organization of implant-supporting elements during the initial healing period [21]. It has been suggested that a practical cut-off value to distinguish between favorable and unfavorable STH should be 2–3 mm in clinical practice [21, 50, 57, 58].

An adequate STH is associated with greater papillary volume and is determined by the connective tissue adhesion level at the adjacent interproximal tooth surface [5, 59, 60]. It is about 3 mm between two adjacent implant restorations, and it is extremely unpredictable and challenging to regenerate [56]. Therefore, an interproximal space morphology should be carefully assessed prior to the implant placement to plan an ideal esthetic outcome [56, 61].

In conclusion, the STH reestablishes an anatomical space for the implant-supporting apparatus, and adequate STH dimension is crucial for long-term peri-implant health. Both functional and esthetic outcomes can be improved by careful examination and possible modification of the STH architecture.

3.5 Peri-Implant Soft Tissue Phenotype Modification and Its Influence on the Long-Term Success of the Implant

Peri-implant phenotype influences the esthetic and functional long-term outcomes of implant treatment [21, 23, 27, 28, 46, 51, 53, 57]. A thin peri-implant mucosa, as measured by the supracrestal tissue height, is correlated with greater marginal bone loss than a thick tissue phenotype [47, 48, 51].

In clinical practice, horizontal and vertical ridge resorption following tooth extraction is commonly observed [62, 63]. Clinicians often perform bone augmentation procedures along with implant surgery; this may induce a coronal displacement of the mucogingival junction, which has a negative effect on peri-implant soft tissue dimension [63, 64]. The following protocols have been suggested as intervention points for soft tissue augmentation: prior to implant placement, at the time of implant surgery, after implant placement but prior to second stage surgery (Fig. 3.4),

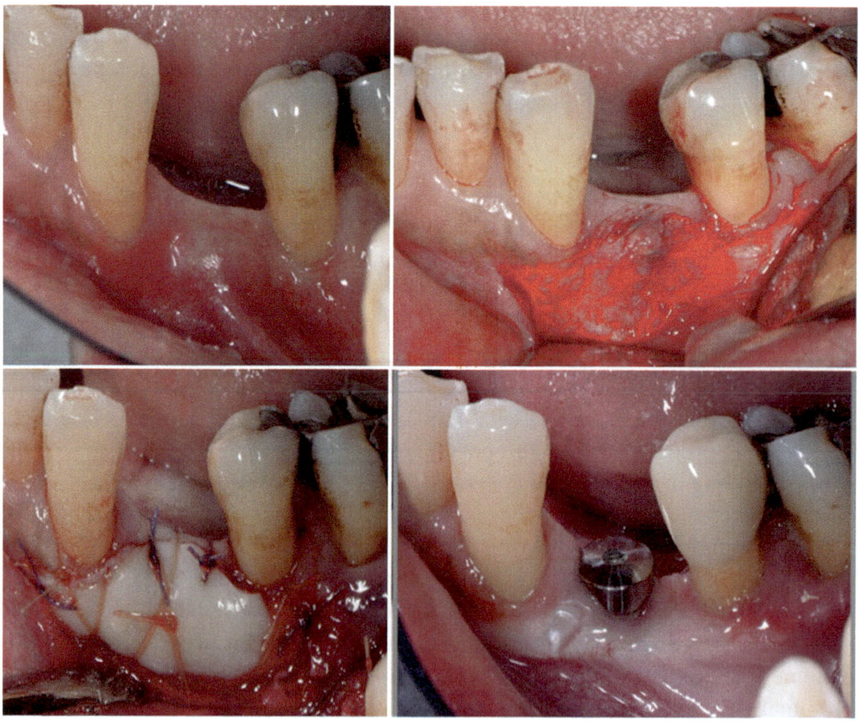

Fig. 3.4 Free gingival graft to increase keratinized gingiva prior to second-stage surgery (Photo courtesy of Dr. Theresa Sun)

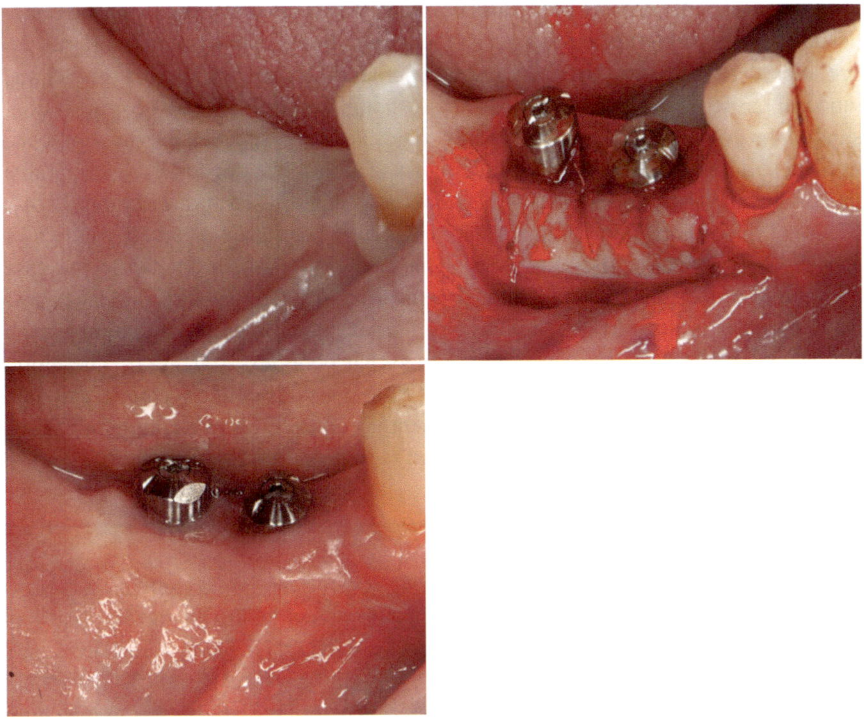

Fig. 3.5 Free gingival graft at the time of second-stage surgery (Photo courtesy of Dr. Giac Dang)

at the time of stage two (implant uncovering) surgery (Fig. 3.5), and after the implant is already uncovered. Intervention after an implant is restored is not recommended unless intervention is required due to peri-implant tissue inflammation [63].

Several techniques to increase the peri-implant soft tissue phenotype, including KMW, MTT, and STH, have been suggested [21, 46, 53]. Autogenous free gingival graft and autogenous connective tissue graft have historically been the first therapy of choice because of their proven efficacy around natural dentition [22, 65]. Free gingival grafts not only increase KMW but also deepen the vestibule during the recipient bed preparation. Due to this additional benefit, the free soft tissue graft technique is the preferred therapy when planning an implant-assisted prosthesis, such as implant-supported overdentures [66]. When using a free gingival tissue graft, an apically positioned flap technique should be employed rather than a bilaminar technique because it has been reported that KMW did not significantly increase following the bilaminar technique with free gingival graft [22, 67]. In a study on dogs, free soft tissue autograft (i.e., free gingival graft) placed at an implant site resulted in a greater KMW gain than an apically positioning flap or xenogenic collagen matrix [66, 68]. Connective tissue grating increases mucosal tissue thickness in addition to supracrestal tissue height [22, 66]. This grafting procedure is particularly helpful because it improves the esthetic outcome as well as peri-implant tissue health [22, 65, 67].

To minimize patient morbidity and eliminate a second surgical site for the donor tissue, different allograft and xenograft techniques are also utilized [22, 67, 69]. An acellular dermal matrix can be used to increase keratinized mucosa width and mucosal tissue thickness [22, 67, 70–72]. Although a connective tissue graft is considered the gold standard for the grafting material of choice when augmenting peri-implant soft tissue, an acellular dermal matrix is reported to accomplish comparable mucosal tissue thickness gain as well as increase supracrestal tissue height [22, 47, 67, 70, 73]. A xenogenic collagen matrix has also been used as an alternative for autogenous connective tissue grafting. This material has been known to increase keratinized mucosal width and mucosal tissue thickness [22, 70–72]. When a bilaminar approach is utilized, peri-implant soft tissue phenotype modification with a xenogenic collagen matrix can stabilize marginal bone levels [22, 74]. Therefore, both allogenic and xenogenic soft tissue grafts are considered adequate and safe alternatives, and they may improve treatment acceptance by reducing patient concerns for donor site discomfort and the need for a second surgical site [66].

3.6 Concluding Remarks

The role of peri-implant soft tissue on the long-term health of the implant has historically been considered somewhat controversial. However, most evidence suggests that a thick peri-implant phenotype, wide band of keratinized mucosa, adequate mucosal tissue thickness, and adequate supracrestal tissue height may reduce peri-implant tissue inflammation and future functional and esthetic complications [17, 56, 66]. Clinicians should carefully examine peri-implant phenotypes when planning implant therapy and, if necessary, should create a favorable peri-implant architecture by employing peri-implant soft tissue phenotype modification.

References

1. Smith DE, Zarb GA. Criteria for success of osseointegrated endosseous implants. J Prosthet Dent. 1989;62:567–72.
2. Proskin HM, Jeffcoat RL, Caitlin A, et al. A meta -analytic approach to determine the state of the science on implant stability. Int J Oral Maxillofac Implants. 2007;22(suppl):11–8.
3. Jung RE, Sailer I, Hammerle CH, et al. In vitro color changes of soft tissues caused by restorative materials. Int J Periodontics Restorative Dent. 2007;27:251–7.
4. Lindhe J, Lang NP, Karring T. The mucosa at teeth and implants. Clin Periodontol Implant Dent. 2008;Chapter 3:71–7.
5. Kan JY, Rungcharassaeng K, Umezu K, et al. Dimensions of peri-implant mucosa: an evaluation of maxillary anterior single implants in humans. J Periodontol. 2003;74:557–62.
6. Lee A, Fu JH, Wang HL. Soft tissue biotype affects implant success. Implant Dent. 2011;20(3):e38–47.
7. Derks J, Hakansson WJL, et al. Effectiveness of implant therapy analyzed in a Swedish population: early and late implant loss. J Dent Res. 2015;94:44S–51S.

8. Cochran DL, Hermann JS, Schenk RK, et al. Biologic width around titanium implants. A histometric analysis of the implant-gingival junction around unloaded and loaded nonsubmerged implants in the canine mandible. J Periodontol. 1997;68:186–98.
9. Sanavi F, Weisgold AS, Rose LF. Biologic width and its relation to periodontal biotypes. J Esthet Dent. 1998;10:157–63.
10. Berglundh T, Lindhe J. Dimension of the peri-implant mucosa. Biological width revisited. J Clin Periodontol. 1996;23:971–3.
11. Berglundh T, Abrahamsson I, Welander M, et al. Morphogenesis of the peri-implant mucosa: an experimental study in dogs. Clin Oral Implants Res. 2007;18:1–8.
12. Abrahamsson I, Berglundh T, Wennstrom J, Lindhe J. The pero-implant hard and soft tissues at different implant systems. A comparative study in dog. Clin Oral Implants Res. 1996;7:212–9.
13. Lindhe J, Berglundhe T. The interface between the mucosa and the implant. Periodontol. 2000;1998(17):47–54.
14. Charpure AS, Latimer JM, Alijofi FE, et al. Role of thin gingival phenotype and inadequate keratoinized mucosa width (<2 mm) as risk indicators for peri-implantitis and peri-implant mucositis. J Periodontol. 2021;92:1–12.
15. Carcuac O, Berglundh T. Composition of human peri-implantitis and periodontitis lesions. J Dent Res. 2015;93:1083–8.
16. Carcuac O, Abrahamsson I, Albouy JP, et al. Experimental periodontitis and peri-implantitis in dog. Clin Oral Implants Res. 2013;24:363–71.
17. Lin GH, Madi IM. Soft tissue biotype affects implant success. Implant Dent. 2011;20(3):138–43.
18. Evans CD, Chen ST. Esthetic outcomes of immediate implant placement. Clin Oral Implants Res. 2008;19:73–80.
19. Bashutski JD, Wang HL. Common implant esthetic complications. Implant Dent. 2007;16:340–8.
20. Lin GH, Chan HL, Wang HL. The significance of keratinized mucosa on implant health: a systemic review. J Periodontol. 2013;84:1755–67.
21. Avila-Ortiz G, Gonzales-Martin O, Couso-Queiruga E, Wang HL. The perio-implant phenotype. J Periodontol. 2020;91(3):283–8.
22. Tavelli L, Barootchi S, Avila-Ortiz G, et al. Peri-implant soft tissue phenotype modification and its impact on peri-implant health: a systematic review and network meta-analysis. J Periodontol. 2021;92:21–44.
23. Arauho MG, Lindhe J. Peri-implant health. J Periodontol. 2018;89(Suppl 1):S249–56.
24. Grischke J, Jarch A, Wernzlaff A, et al. Keratinized mucosa width is associated with severity of peri-implant mucositis. A cross-sectional study. J Clin Oral IMlnt Res. 2019;30:457–65.
25. Monje A, Blasi G. Significance of keratinized mucosa/gingiva on peri-implant and adjacent periodontal conditions in erratic maintenance compliers. J Periodontol. 2019;90:445–53.
26. Perussolo J, Siuza AB, Matarazzo F, et al. Influence of the keratinized mucosa on the stability of peri-implant tissues and brushing discomfort: a 4-year follow up study. Clin Oral Implants Res. 2018;29:1177–85.
27. Bouri A Jr, Bissada N, A-Zahrani MS, et al. Width of keratinized gingiva and the health status of the supporting tissues around dental implants. Int J Oral Maxillofac Implants. 2008;23:323–6.
28. Schou S, Holmstrup P, Hjorting-Hansen E, Lang NP. Plaque-induced marginal tissue reactions of osseointegrated oral implants: a review of the literature. Clin Oral Implants Res. 1992;3:149–61.
29. Wennstrom JL, Derks J. Is there a need for keratinized mucosa around implants to maintain health and tissue stability? Clin Oral Implants Res. 2012;23(Suppl 6):136–46.
30. Adibrad M, Shahabuei M, Sahabi M. Significance of the width of keratinized mucosa on the health status of the supporting overdentures. J Oral Implantol. 2009;35:232–7.
31. Roccuzzo M, Grasso G, Dalmasso P. Keratinized mucosa around implants in partially edentulous posterior mandible: 10-year results of a prospective comparative study. Clin Oral Implants Res. 2016;27:491–6.

32. Zigdon H, Machtei EE. The dimensions of keratinized mucosa around implants affect clinical and immunological parameters. Clin Oral Implants Res. 2008;19(4):387–91.
33. Chung DM, Oh TJ, Shotwell JL, et al. Significance of keratinized mucosa in maintenance of dental implants with different surfaces. J Periodontol. 2006;77(8):1410–20.
34. Schwartz F, Derks J, Monje A, Wang HL. Peri-implantitis. J Clin Periodontol. 2018;45(Suppl):S246–66.
35. Gobatto L, Avila-Ortiz G, Sohrabi K, et al. The effect of keratinized mucosa width on peri-implant health: a systemic review. Int J Oral Maxillofac Implants. 2013;28(6):1536–45.
36. Crespi R, Cappare P, Ghelone E. A 4-year evaluation of the peri-implant parameters of immediately loaded implants placed in fresh extraction sockets. J Periodontol. 2010;81(11):1629–34.
37. Brito C, Tenenbaum HC, Wong BKC, et al. Is keratinized mucosa indispensable to maintain peri-implant health? A systemic review of the literature. J Biomed Mater Res B Appl Biomater. 2014;102B:643–50.
38. Kim BS, Kim TK, Yun PY, et al. Evaluation of peri-implant tissue response according to the presence of keratinized mucosa. Oral Surg Oral Med Oral Pathol Oral Radiol Endod. 2009;107(3):e24–8.
39. Warrer K, Buser D, Lang NP, Karring T. Plaque-induced peri-implantitis in the presence or absence of keratinized mucosa: an experimental study in monkeys. Clin Oral Implants Res. 1995;6:131–8.
40. Roos-Jansaker AM, Renvert H, Lindahl C, Renvert S. Nine to fourteen year follow-up of implant treatment. Part III: factors associated with peri-implant lesions. J Clin Periodontol. 2006;33:296–301.
41. Greenstein G, Cavallaro J. The clinical significance of keratinized gingiva around dental implants. Compend Contin Educ Dent. 2011;32(8):24–31.
42. Wang HL, Zucchelli G. Significance of peri-implant keratinized mucosa width and soft tissue thickness. Int J Periodont Rest Dent. 2019;39(6):767–8.
43. Cosyn J, Sabzevar MM, De Bruyn H. Predictors of inter-proximal and midfacial recession following single implant treatment in the anterior maxilla: a multivariate analysis. J Clin Periodontol. 2012;39:895–903.
44. Park SE, Da Silva JD, Weber HP, Ishikawa-Nagai S. Optical phenomenon of peri-implant soft tissue. Part I. Spectrophotometric assessment of natural tooth gingiva and peri-implant mucosa. Clin Oral Implants Res. 2007;18:569–74.
45. Kim A, Campbell SD, Viana MA, Knoernschild KL. Abutment material effect on peri-implant soft tissue color and perceived esthetics. J Prosthodont. 2016;25:634–40.
46. Lops S, Stellini E, Sbricoli L, et al. Influence of abutment material on peri-implant soft tissues in anterior areas with thin gingival biotype; a multicentric prospective study. Clin Oral Implants Res. 2017;28:1263–8.
47. Puisys A, Linkevicius T. The influence of mucosal tissue thickening on crestal bone stability around bone -level implants. A prospective controlled clinical trial. Clin Oral Implants Res. 2015;26:123–9.
48. Linkevicius T, Apse P, Grybauskas S, Puisys A. The influence of soft tissue thickness on crestal bone changes around implants: a 1-year prospective controlled clinical trial. Int J Oral Maxillofac Implants. 2009;24:712–9.
49. Dibart S, Warbington M, Su MF, Skobe Z. In vitro evaluation of the implant-abutment bacterial seal: the locking taper system. Int J Oral Maxillofac Implants. 2005;20:732–7.
50. Suarez-Lopez del Amo F, Lin G, Monje A, et al. Influence of soft tissue thickness on peri-implant marginal bone loss: a systemic review and meta-analysis. J Periodontol. 2016;87(6):690–8.
51. Linkevicius T, Puisys A, Linkeviciene L, et al. Crestal bone stability around implants with horizontally matching connection after soft tissue thickening: a prospective clinical trial. Clin Implant Dent Res. 2015;17:497–508.

52. Weisner G, Esposito M, Worthington H, Schlee M. Connective tissue grafts for thickening peri-implant tissues at implant placement. One-year results from an explanatory split-mouth randomized controlled clinical trial. Eur J Oral Implantol. 2010;3:27–35.
53. Thoma DS, Naenni N, Figuero E, et al. Effects of soft tissue augmentation procedures on peri-implant health or disease; a systemic review and meta-analysis. Clin Oral Implants Res. 2018;29(suppl 15):32–49.
54. Yoshino S, Kan JY, Rungcharassaeng K, et al. Effects of connective tissue grafting on the facial gingival level following single immediate implant placement and provisionalization in the esthetic zone: a 1-year randomized controlled prospective study. Int J Oral Maxillofac Implants. 2014;29:432–40.
55. Magliorati M, Amorfini L, Signori A, et al. Clinical and aesthetic outcome with post-extractive implants with or without soft tissue augmentation; a 2-year randomized clinical trial. Clin Implant Dent Relat Res. 2015;17:983–95.
56. Wang I, Barootchi S, Tavelli WH. The peri-implant phenotype and implant esthetic complications. Contemporary overview. J Esthet Restor Dent. 2021;33:212–23.
57. Linkevicius T, Linkevivius R, Alkimavicius J, et al. Influence of titanium base, lithium disilicate restoration and vertical soft tissue thickness on bone stability around triangular-shaped implants: a prospective clinical trial. Clin Oral Implants Res. 2018;29:716–24.
58. Diaz-Sanchez M, Soto-Penaloza D, Penarrocha-Oltra D, Penarrocha-Diago M. Influence of supracrestal tissue attachment thickness on radiographic bone level around dental implants: a systemic review and meta-analysis. J Periodontal Res. 2019;54:573–88.
59. Zweers J, Thomas R, Slot D, et al. Characteristics of periodontal biotype, its dimensions, associations, and prevalence: a systemic review. J Clin Periodontol. 2014;41:958–71.
60. Palmer R, Farknodeh N, Palmer P, Wilson R. Astra tech single-tooth implants: an audit of patient satisfaction and soft tissue form. J Clin Periodontol. 2007;34:633–8.
61. Roccuzzo M, Roccuzzo A, Ramanuskaite A. Papilla height in relation to the distance between bone crest and interproximal contact point at single-tooth implants: a systemic review. Clin Oral Implants Res. 2018;29(15):50–61.
62. Araujo MG, LIndhe J. Ridge alterations following tooth extraction with and without flap elevation: an experimental study in the dog. Clin Oral Implants Res. 2009;20:545–9.
63. Bassetti M, Kaufmann R, Salivi GE, et al. Soft tissue grafting to improve the attached mucosa at dental implants: a review of the literature and proposal of a decision tree. Quintessence Int. 2015;46(6):499–50.
64. Stimmelmayr M, Allen EP, Reichert TE, Iglhaut G. Use of a combination epithelized subepithelial connective tissue graft for closure and soft tissue augmentation of an extraction site following ridge preservation or implant placement: description of a technique. Int J Periodontics Restorative Dent. 2010;30:375–81.
65. Zucchelli G, Tavelli L, McGuire MK, et al. Autogenous soft tissue grafting for periodontal and peri-implant plastic surgical reconstruction. J Periodontol. 2020;91:9–16.
66. Saitz AE. Impact of keratinized mucosa in dental implant treatment. Decis Dent. 2020;6(8):40–4.
67. Tavelli L, McGuire MK, Zucchelli G, et al. Extracellular matrix based scaffolding technologies for periodontal and peri-implant soft tissue regeneration. J Periodontol. 2020;91:17–25.
68. Thoma D, Lim H, Paeng K, et al. Augmentation of keratinized tissue at tooth and implant sites by using autogenous grafts and collagen-based soft-tissue substitutes. J Clin Periodontol. 2020;47:64–71.
69. Tavelli L, Ravida A, Saleh M, et al. Pain perception following epithelialized gingival grafting harvesting: a randomized clinical trial. Clin Oral Investig. 2019;23:459–68.
70. Tavelli L, Barootchi S, Di Gianfillippo R, et al. Acellular dermal matrix and coronally advanced flap or tunnel technique in the treatment of multiple adjacent gingival recessions. A 12-year follow-up from a randomized clinical trial. J Clin Periodontol. 2019;46:937–48.

71. Ahmedbeyli C, Ipci SD, Cakar G, et al. Clinical evaluation of coronally advanced flap with without acellular dermal matrix graft on complete defect coverage for the treatment of multiple gingival recessions with thin tissue biotype. J Clin Periodontol. 2014;41:303–10.
72. De Queiroz CA, Sallum AW, Casati MZ, et al. A two-year prospective study of coronally positioned flap with or without acellular dermal matrix graft. J Clin Periodontol. 2006;33:683–9.
73. Puisys A, Vindasiute E, Linkevciene L, Linkevciene T. The use of acellular dermal matrix membrane for vertical soft tissue augmentation during submerged implant placement; a case series. Clin Oral Implants Res. 2015;26:465–70.
74. Thoma DS, Gasser T, Jung RE, Hammerle C. Randomized controlled clinical trial comparing implant sites augmented with a volume-stable collagen matrix or an autogenous connective tissue graft: 3-year data after insertion of reconstructions. J Clin Periodontol. 2020;47:630–9.

Soft Tissue Management During Different Stage of Surgical Placement of Dental Implants

4

Mohamed Hassan

4.1 Introduction

Dental implants are now considered the gold standard for replacing missing teeth. Recent advancements in technology have significantly increased the success rate of dental implants.

In a 10-year retrospective study, it was found that the implant survival rate is 98.8% and there is a success rate of 97.0%. In addition, the prevalence of peri-implantitis in this large cohort of orally healthy patients was low at 1.8% during the 10-year period [1].

Due to that high success rate, it is estimated that between 300,000–428,000 dental implants are placed every year in the USA [2].

This high success rate encouraged more patients to consider dental implants as the preferred option when determining their treatment plan. With the wide use of dental implants, it has become essential more than ever to ensure short- and long-term success and satisfactory results for both clinicians and patients.

The success of dental implants is determined by multiple factors, some of which are related to the clinicians' ability to achieve optimum results and collaboration with other dental care providers. Other factors are related to the patient's medical and dental conditions and their level of compliance with the dental healthcare providers' instructions and guidelines. However, it is worth noting that the success rate could be increased by altering some factors related to the patient's condition, such as smoking secession, appliance therapy to manage parafunctions, and improving oral hygiene measures.

M. Hassan (✉)
Oral Medicine, Infection & Immunity, Harvard School of Dental Medicine, Boston, MA, USA
e-mail: Mohamed_Hassan@hsdm.harvard.edu

M. Hassan (ed.), *Peri-Implant Soft Tissue Management*,
https://doi.org/10.1007/978-3-031-45516-2_4

Dental practitioners are advised to carefully analyze all factors before considering the placement of implants to restore edentulous space and do their best to ensure proper requirements for reasonably predicted successful procedures.

Due to the increased demand for the use of dental implants as an accepted modality to replace missing teeth, more dentists are involved in the surgical phase of dental implants.

In order to achieve more successful results in dental implants, dental practitioners who decide to incorporate dental implants as a modality in their practice are required to have adequate theoretical and clinical knowledge of the properties and biomechanics of implants. In addition, they should understand the properties of surrounding tissues and correction methods to avoid failure. Using dental implants to replace missing teeth without this adequate knowledge may lead to ethical, legal, and moral challenges due to avoidable complications and failures.

These failures can result in pain and suffering by patients and complicated, time-consuming, and costly procedures to rectify the problems, which still may not guarantee positive outcomes. Dental implants are surrounded in the oral cavity by two types of tissues: hard and soft tissues. Both tissues are affected after tooth extraction, which may pose a challenge during both surgical and restorative phases of implant dentistry. It is estimated that after extraction, up to 50% of the width of the bone may be lost. Such bone loss will lead to coronal displacement of the mucogingival junction. This may necessitate one or more additional corrective surgical procedures [3].

These surgical interventions may be incorporated into different phases of the surgical or restorative treatment to achieve the desired optimum successful results. Improving the quality and quantity of both types of tissues depends on each other. While bone structure is essential to provide a healthy foundation for implant stability, it is also important to maintain healthy and adequate overlying soft tissues to ensure long term aesthetic and functional satisfactory results. As a result of resorption or remodeling of the surrounding housing bony structures, keratinized mucosa may also be deficient, which will negatively impact implant placement afterward [4].

On the other hand, the presence of thin alveolar mucosa will lead to a higher alveolar buccal bony resorption and more apical tissues marginal position during implant placement regardless of the thickness of the buccal bony crest [5]. Hence, it is recommended to improve the quantity and quality of soft tissues surrounding the implant to ensure proper bony support for dental implant.

Se-Lim et al. examined the crestal bone loss around implants following the free gingival graft group in comparison to a control group that shows a lack of keratinized mucosa. They found that crestal bone loss is significantly greater in the control group than in the individual with adequate keratinized mucosa after soft tissue augmentation during 18 months study [6]. In another study by Warrer K et al., in which they examined the importance of adequate healthy keratinized mucosa around ligated implants in monkeys, they found that lack of proper width of keratinized mucosa will lead to more soft tissue recession, greater loss of attachment, and increased depth of angular bony defect [7]. In addition, the width of the keratinized tissues influences immunological parameters [8, 9].

The need for keratinized mucosa is still a controversial matter and is disputed in the literature [10–13]. Lang and Loe reported that teeth with less than 2 mm of KT may exhibit more gingival inflammation and gingival exudate despite the plaque-free surface of teeth [14]. Other studies found that even with the lack of keratinized tissues around teeth, it is possible to maintain healthy gingival tissues around teeth [15, 16].

It was concluded that in order to maintain a healthy periodontium, it is recommended to have at least 2 mm or more of keratinized tissues around natural dentition. Soft tissues surrounding natural teeth are structurally and anatomically different than those around dental implants. Tissues around natural dentition can be categorized into keratinized and nonkeratinized oral mucosa. Meanwhile, peri-implant soft tissues are still inconsistently described in the literature [17]. A dental implant does not have periodontal ligament space, which decreases the amount of blood supply [18].

Also, there is an anatomical difference between the direction of connective tissue fibers around the implant versus natural teeth as follows (implants = parallel, teeth = perpendicular) [19, 20]. Due to the nature of keratinized tissues, it is assumed that it would help prevent bacterial penetration and allow proper oral hygiene measures to be performed, which is essential for long-term success [21]. Adequate keratinized mucosa will allow maintenance to be performed without the patient's discomfort [22]. Keratinized mucosa will also decrease plaque accumulation [23] and decrease the possibility of gingival recession and tissue inflammation around dental implants [24]. Because of the wide range of documented evidence of the importance of the presence of a collar-like band of keratinized mucosa, it is reasonable to think it is important to have at least a minimum of 2 mm of healthy keratinized gingiva around dental implants. In the case of the absence of a minimal amount, dental practitioners should consider augmenting the deficient gingival tissues to ensure long-term accepted functional and aesthetic outcomes.

Soft tissue augmentation around dental implants can be addressed at different times using different techniques. The attached gingiva (AG) is that portion of gingiva that extends from the base of the gingival crevice to the mucogingival junction. According to the glossary of periodontal terms, AG is firm, resilient, and tightly bound to the underlying periosteum of alveolar bone through connective tissue. To augment peri-implant soft tissues, two methods can be considered. One option is to increase the width of keratinized mucosa by using an apically positioned flap with or without a gingival graft. The second option is to increase the volume gain by means of a sub-epithelial connective tissue graft in the case of a thin biotype [25]. Both techniques are proven to have a positive impact on the long-term stability of the peri-implant soft tissues and increase the predictability of implant therapy over time [24, 26–30].

Soft tissue deficiencies can be corrected during different phases of the surgical or restorative stage of dental implant treatment. They may be corrected before placement, during placement, during the second stage phase, or sometimes after loading the implants [31]. Most studies recommend performing corrective surgeries before starting the restorative phase to avoid complications such as mucositis and peri-implantitis [17, 32, 33].

Identifying the etiology of the defect is essential for successful correction. The sources of the defect may include patient-related factors such as smoking, poor oral hygiene, or immunocompromised status. Anatomy-related factors include gingival biotype, flap thickness and defect depth, height, and width. Procedure-related variations include surgically implemented techniques and practitioners' surgical abilities [34].

This chapter reviews different techniques and timing for correcting soft tissue deficiencies to achieve proper esthetic and functional outcomes. Although most techniques for soft tissue correction can be implemented and applied during different phases, some of which may need to be modified to serve certain purposes during a particular phase. Collaboration between dental care providers plays an integral role in helping deliver the best results during all phases of implant dentistry. During the planning phase, a complete and comprehensive evaluation is essential to apply the proper technique at a certain stage.

4.2 Before Surgical Placement of Implants

Tissue regeneration, whether hard or soft, can be addressed before starting the surgical phase of implant placement. Having a long-standing edentulous area may lead to deficiencies of hard and soft tissues, with both affecting each other. Regeneration of one type can be influenced by the adequate presence of the other. Surgical procedures will lead to the formation of scar tissues, which may complicate soft tissue handling for future surgeries [35]. Scar tissues manifest less elasticity than mucosal tissues. Elasticity is required to achieve primary closure for GBR, especially vertical augmentation for complete coverage for the grafted bone. Incorporating more than one surgical procedure will decrease the frequency of surgeries and scar tissue formation. In case soft tissue correction is required, dental practitioners may implement different techniques to increase the zone of attached gingiva before starting implant placement.

4.2.1 Free Gingival Graft

First described by Sullivan and Atkins (1968) [36], the free gingival graft is considered one of the most common procedures utilized to increase the width and thickness of keratinized mucosa around natural teeth and dental implants. FGG is utilized to prevent or manage keratinized gingiva inadequacy. Careful pre-surgical evaluation is essential due to the limitation of the amount that can be harvested from the donor site [37]. As Harvey in 1970 recommended, it takes the recipient site approximately 6 months before undergoing another surgical procedure [38]. Postoperative pain [39] and bleeding are considered common disadvantages of the FGG procedure. Despite the well-known disadvantages, FGG is still considered the gold standard for soft tissue augmentation. Because of the known disadvantages, soft tissue substitutes were introduced and utilized to replace FGG. Even though they offer less postoperative pain and discomfort and solve the problem of limited autogenous tissue supply, the outcome is still inferior to that of FGG. Shrinkage and inconsistent quality of the generated soft tissues are considered major limitations, which may limit the implementation of FGG substitutes [40]. Furthermore, acellular dermal matrix (ADM) may result in regenerated tissues resembling scar tissues [41].

4.2.1.1 Before Teeth Extraction

As mentioned earlier, long-standing edematous areas may result in both hard and soft tissue insufficiency. The following case describes a female patient using a removable partial denture supported on the hopeless remaining mandibular anterior dentition. The patient is interested in having an implant-supported complete denture. Clinical and radiographic evaluation shows severe loss of both hard and soft tissues. FGG was indicated to increase the amount of keratinized gingival tissues and allow for primary closure during vertical bone augmentation. Hard and soft tissue augmentation will provide enough support for the dental implants. To minimize the needed surgical procedures and necessary time required to complete the case, combining more than one surgery in the same setting is recommended if possible.

To achieve the goals in this case, a free soft tissue graft was performed during the extraction procedure, as shown in Figs. 4.1, 4.2, 4.3, and 4.4.

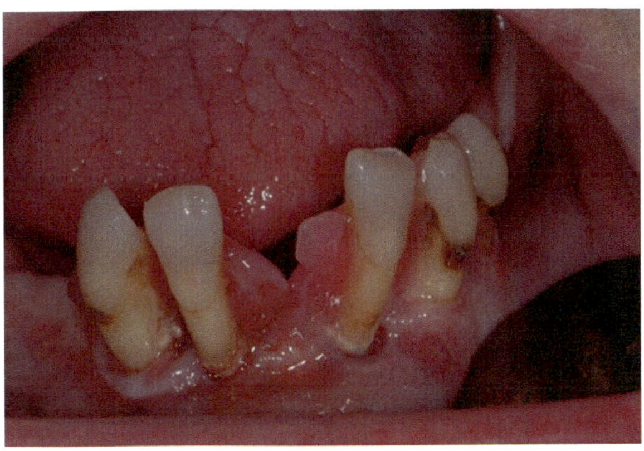

Fig. 4.1 Remaining anterior dentition with denture adhesive

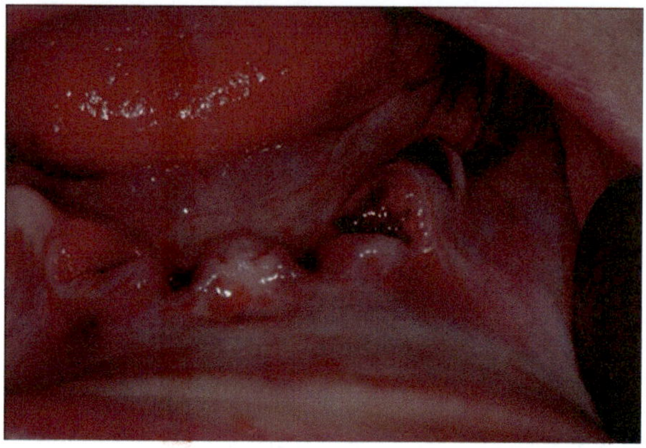

Fig. 4.2 After extraction of mandibular dentition

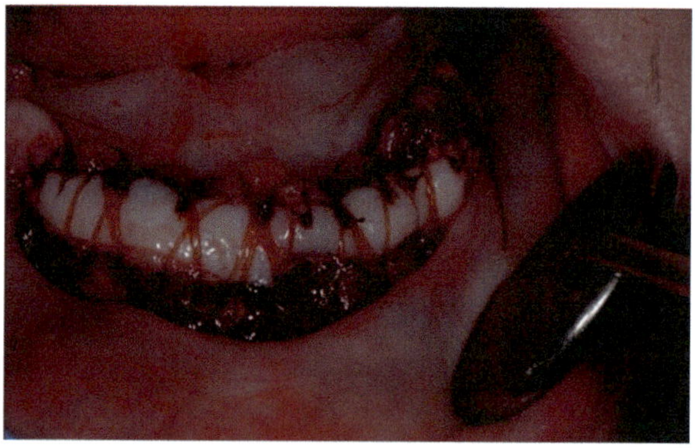

Fig. 4.3 Free soft tissue graft

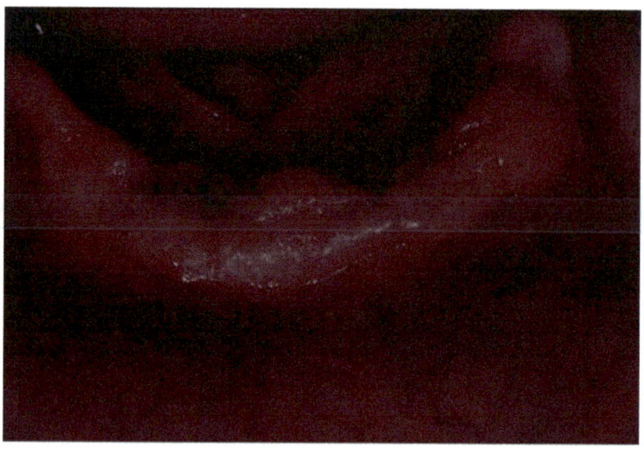

Fig. 4.4 Healing after free soft tissue graft

4.2.1.2 After Teeth Extraction

A completely edentulous patient has a treatment plan to have implant-supported complete dentures. The success of implants is questionable due to a significant lack of hard and soft tissues. Soft tissue augmentation may take place first, as shown in Figs. 4.5 and 4.6. Once completed, soft tissue augmentation will be followed by hard tissue regeneration before considering implant placement, as shown in Figs. 4.7, 4.8, and 4.9.

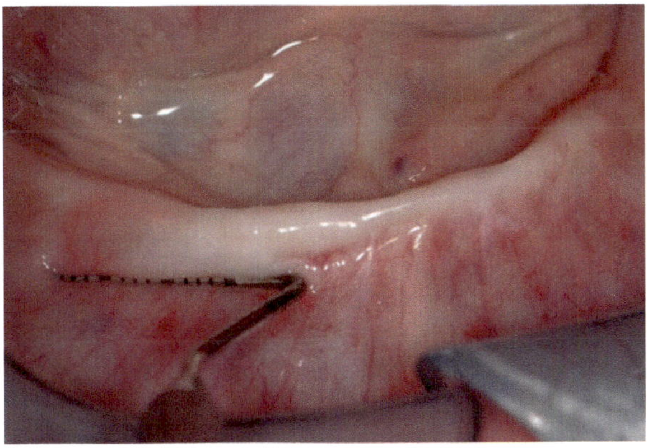

Fig. 4.5 Severe lack of hard and soft tissues

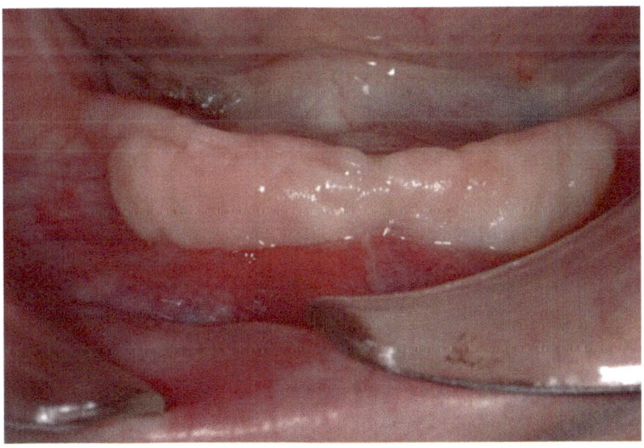

Fig. 4.6 After soft tissue graft to increase zone of keratinized gingiva

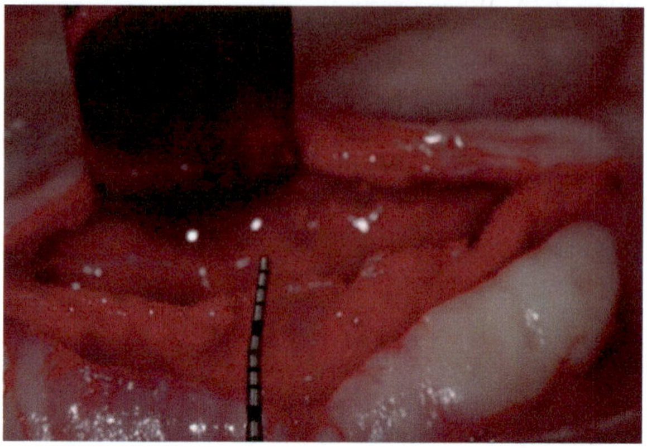

Fig. 4.7 Hard tissue augmentation

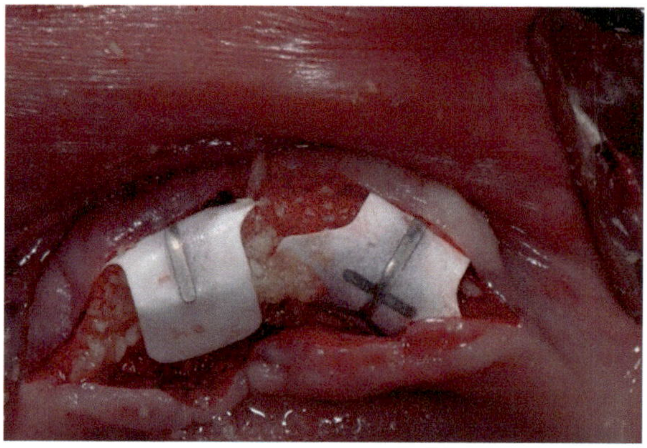

Fig. 4.8 Bone grafting

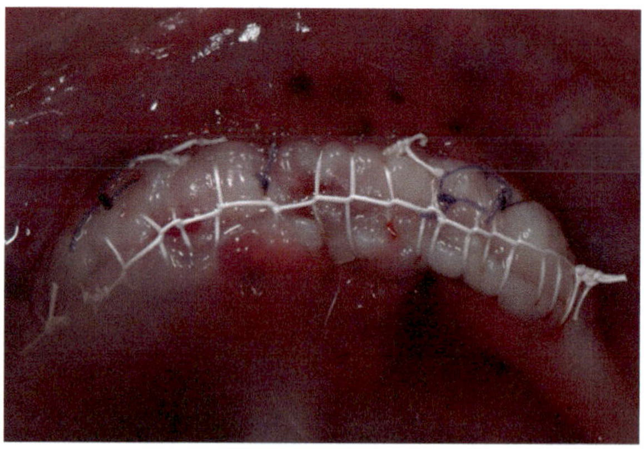

Fig. 4.9 Soft tissue augmentation allowed for primary closure

4.3 During Surgical Placement of Implants

Quality and quantity of soft tissues can be maintained and protected by implementing proper flap design during the surgical procedure. Proper technique will offer different advantages while imposing some restrictions. Dentists need to make a sound decision on which design to apply to achieve the desired goals of a specific procedure. Flap design plays an essential role in providing proper access while maintaining the soft tissues' integrity. This will result in proper outcomes both aesthetically and functionally. Any flap design should fulfill the basic flap requirement and provide the following [42]:

1. Optimal visualization.
2. Problem-free expansion of the soft tissues.
3. Mobilization of the overlying soft tissue to cover the surgical field.
4. No placement over bony defects or cavities.
5. Sufficient vascularization of soft tissue.
6. Minimum esthetic impairment and good tissue covering.

Regardless of the flap design, the healing process will result in scaring formation, which impacts esthetic and functional outcomes. Blood supply in the surgical area must be maintained at a sufficient level during different surgical stages. Kleinheinz et al. in 2005 described the proper incisions during flap reflection to minimize blood supply interruption at the surgical site in order to prevent complications, as shown in Fig. 4.10a–c. An avascular mid-crestal incision seems to be the ideal choice in the edentulous area and to restrict the application of a vertical releasing incision to the anterior end of the flap. Blood vessels run from the posterior to anterior area. Positioning the vertical incision anteriorly will prevent blood supply interruption. A trapezoid flap should be avoided if adequate access can be achieved by anterior vertical releasing incision only. The color of gingival tissues depends on the blood vessels and tissues' keratinization; less keratinization and more blood vessels will yield more red color and vice versa [43].

During the surgical phase, implants can be placed utilizing either the flapped or flapless surgical approach. A flapped technique provides a better soft tissue emergence profile as it allows the surgeon to place the soft tissue in the proper desired contour [44]. A flapless technique is a minimally invasive approach that helps maintain blood supply and avoid interruption of blood flow to the surgical site while providing limited access to the surgical site. The flapped technique provides better visibility through a full-thickness mucoperiosteal flap. The full-thickness flap helps protect and identify anatomical landmarks [45] with the disadvantage of causing blood supply interruption to the surgical field. Blood supply interruption will lead to crestal bone resorption and some long-term esthetic and functional complications. The flapped technique is still the approach of choice in case bone augmentation is indicated to compensate for hard tissue deficiencies.

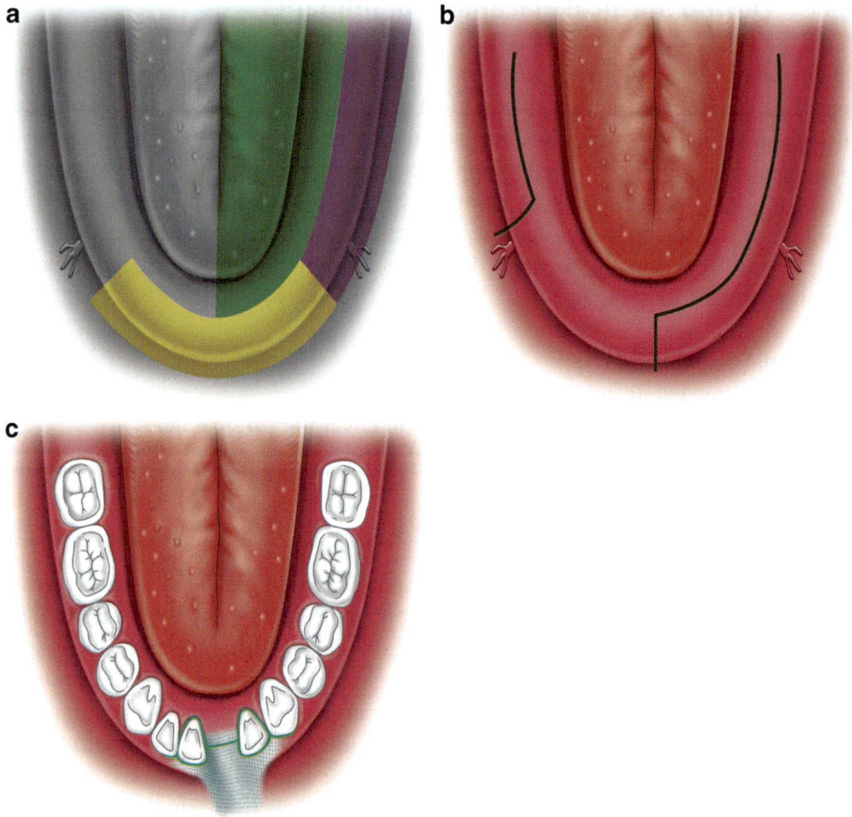

Fig. 4.10 (**a**) Displays the midcrestal incision line, while (**b**) shows the proper position for vertical releasing incision, and (**c**) illustrates the proper envelop flap design

4.3.1 Flap Technique

Figure 4.11 shows a patient with missing tooth #26. Due to the inadequacy of interdental space shown in Fig. 4.11, the patient has undergone orthodontic treatment to provide enough space for proper implant-supported crown restoration to prevent space loss.

After completing the course of orthodontic treatment, as shown in Figs. 4.12 and 4.13, the patient presented to pursue implant placement. A treatment plan was developed with immediate loading of the implant as a space maintainer to guard

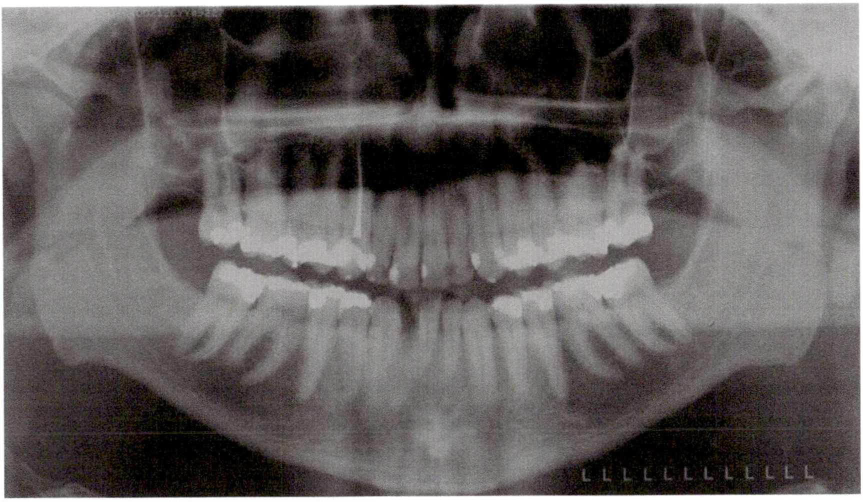

Fig. 4.11 Panoramic x-ray before othodontic intervention

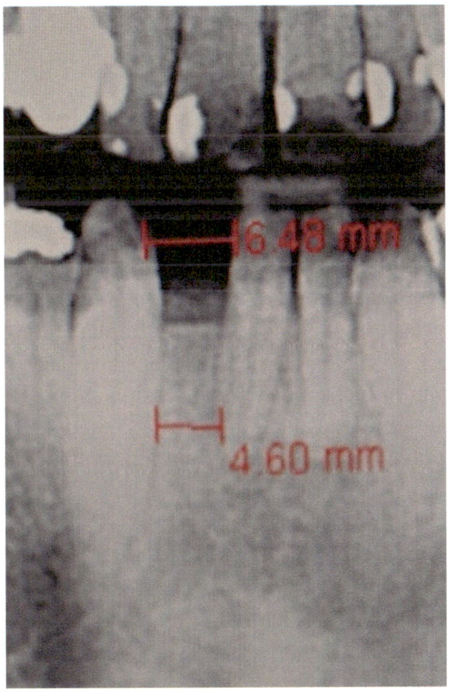

Fig. 4.12 Radiograph after orthodontic treatment was completed

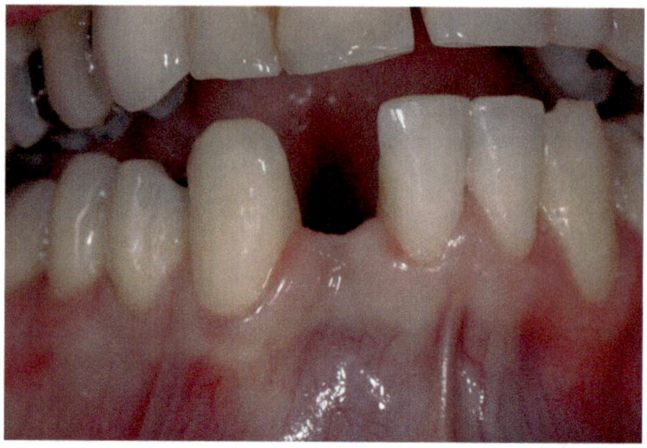

Fig. 4.13 Clinical image after orthodontic treatment

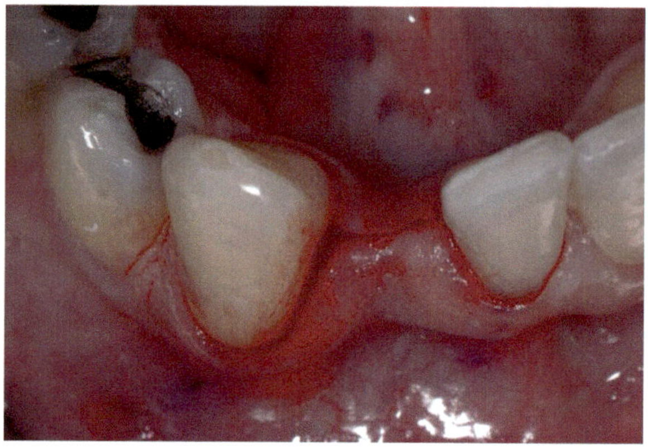

Fig. 4.14 Proper flap design described by Kleinheinz et al

against space loss. In addition, this approach allows the patient not to use a retainer after orthodontic treatment. Implementing the Kleinheinz flap design as shown in Fig. 4.14, an implant was placed with hard tissue augmentation and immediate loading in the same surgical session (Figs. 4.15, 4.16, 4.17, 4.18, and 4.19). Five-year follow-up evaluation (Figs. 4.20 and 4.21) show stable functional and esthetic outcomes, both clinically and radiographically.

4.3.2 Flapless Technique

A patient with a missing mandibular anterior dentition presented for implant placement. The treatment consists of replacing missing dentitions with implant-supported fixed partial dentures.

Utilizing the flapless technique provides intact mucoperiosteum, which offers advantages such as less bleeding, less postoperative pain, rapid postoperative healing, and less surgical time [46–48]. Disadvantages include the possibility of hard tissue perforation and/or fenestration due to lack of visibility, which may also cause

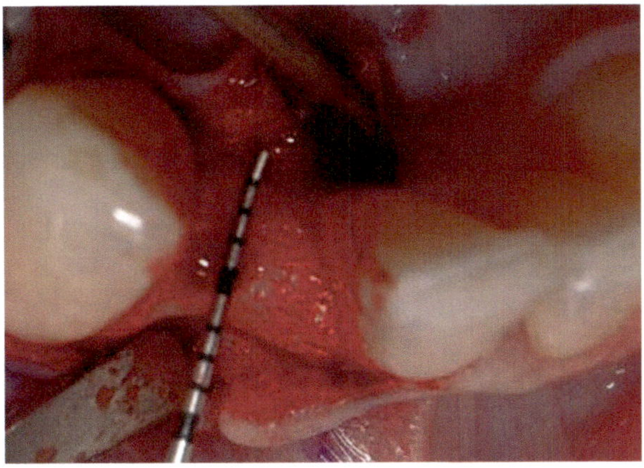

Fig. 4.15 Proper flap design allows for accessibility

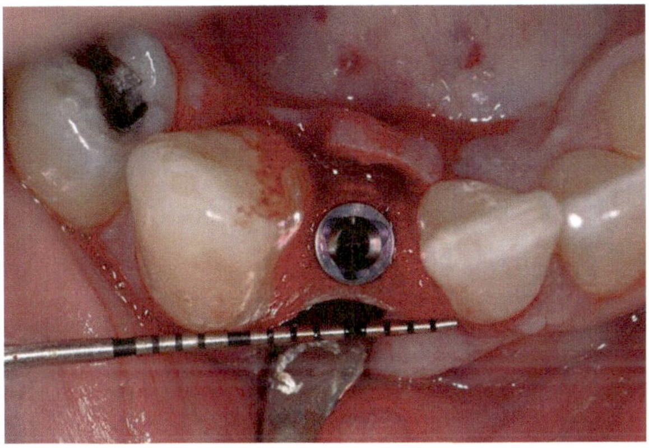

Fig. 4.16 After implant placement shows the need for hard tissue augmentation

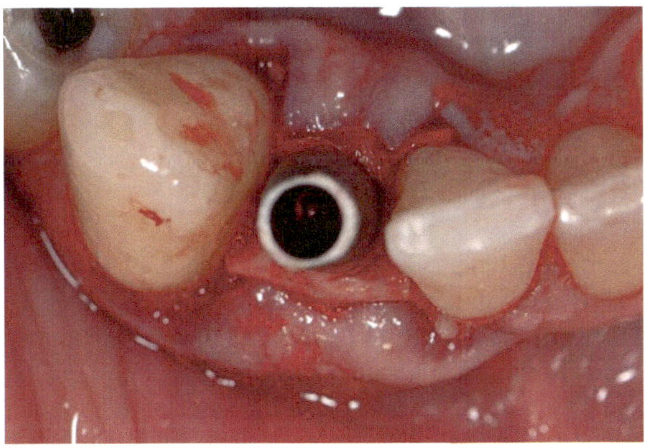

Fig. 4.17 Hard tissue augmentation and temporary abutment

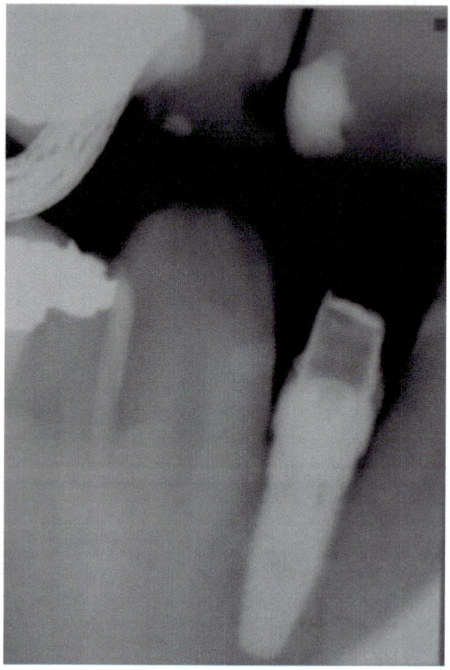

Fig. 4.18 Periapical x-ray immediately after implant placement

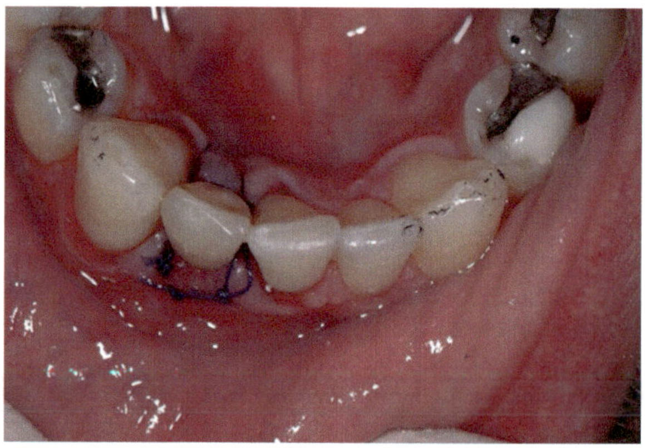

Fig. 4.19 Immediate loading

anatomical landmark threats [49]. The flapless technique should be restricted to cases with anticipated adequate width and height of bone and soft tissues. Figures 4.22, 4.23, 4.24, and 4.25 show extraction of hopeless teeth #22–27 followed by bone augmentation and implant placement in the area of missing teeth #22 and 27. Figures 4.26 and 4.27 show implant-supported fixed partial dentures replacing extracted teeth #22–27.

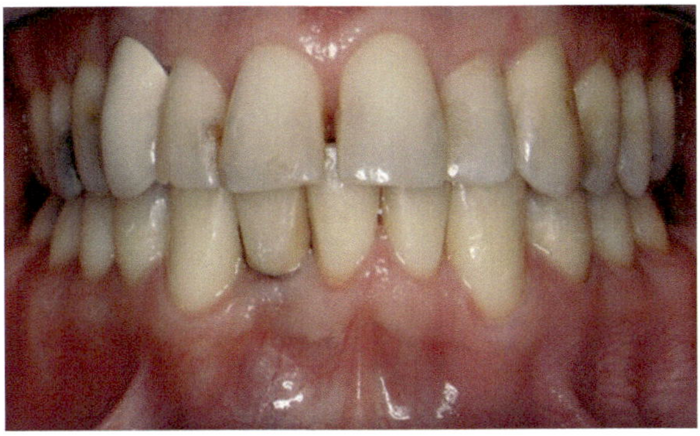

Fig. 4.20 Five-year follow up

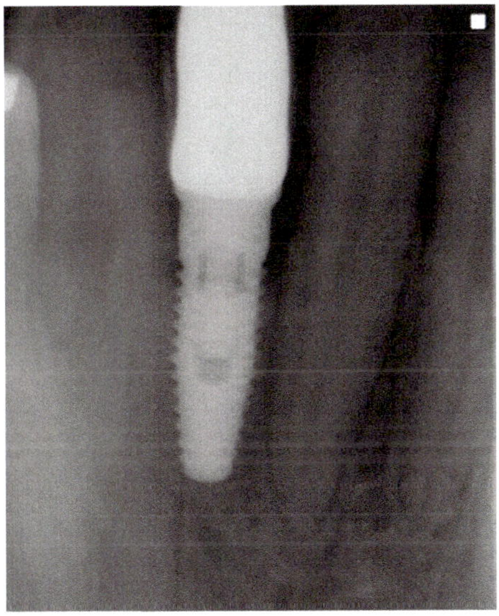

Fig. 4.21 Five-year periapical x-ray

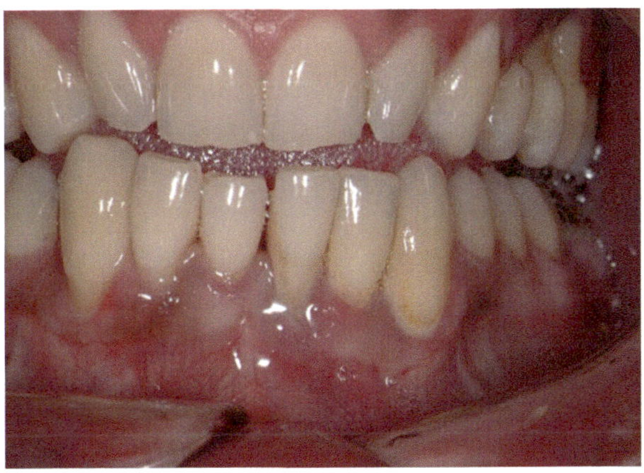

Fig. 4.22 Hopeless teeth #23–27

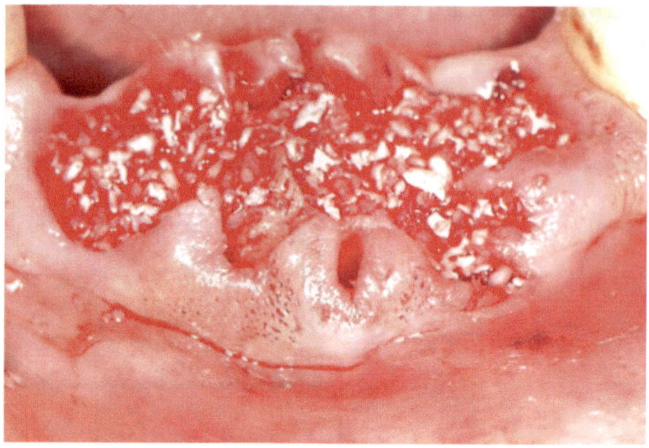

Fig. 4.23 Bone augmentation to prepare for implant placement

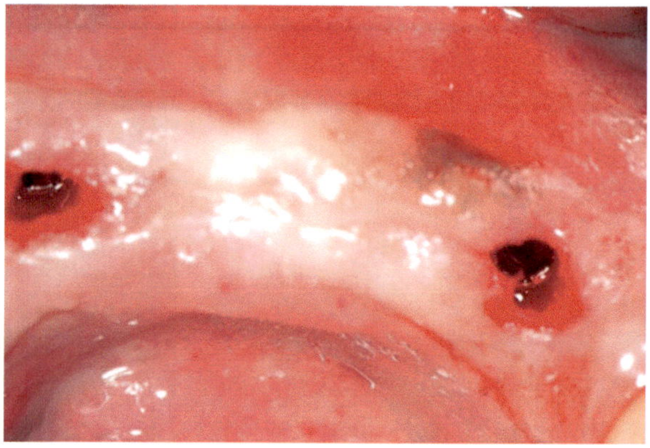

Fig. 4.24 Flapless implant placement

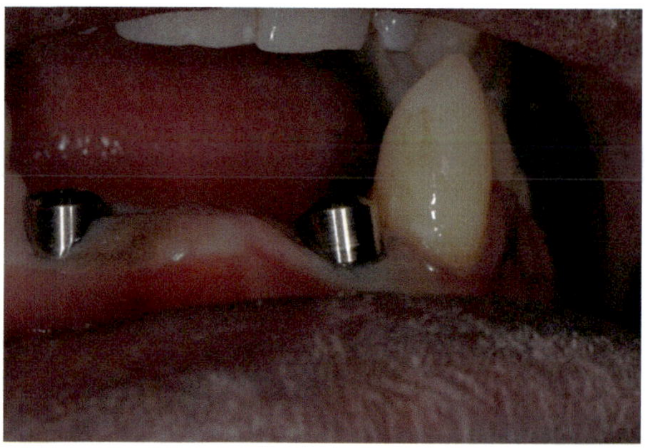

Fig. 4.25 One-stage immediate implant placement

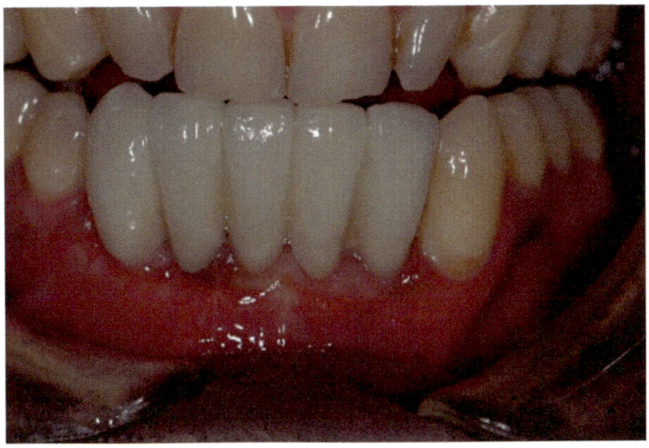

Fig. 4.26 Implant-supported fixed partial denture

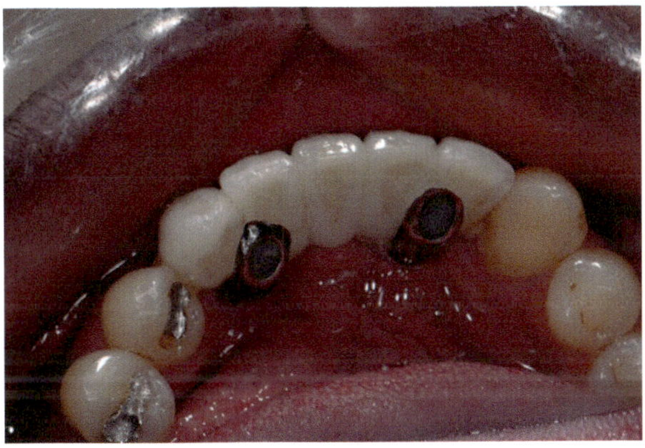

Fig. 4.27 Implant-supported fixed partial denture

4.4 During Second Stage

Soft tissue deficiencies can be corrected during the second stage of implant surgery. This section of the chapter reviews different techniques that can be utilized to address such problems. The dentist should use clinical judgment to determine which technique, classical or modified, would best match the clinical circumstances and to provide better aesthetic and/or functional outcomes.

4.4.1 Apically Positioning Flap

An apically positioned flap is a simple modality to increase the zone of keratinized tissues around natural teeth and dental implants. This technique does not involve a second surgical site as in free gingival and connective tissue grafts. One of the limitations of this technique, though, is that it does not increase biotype thickness (Figs. 4.28, 4.29, and 4.30).

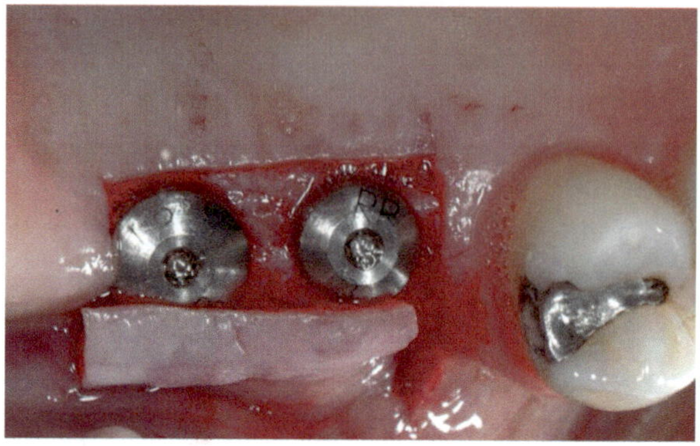

Fig. 4.28 Increasing zone of keratinized gingiva around dental implants

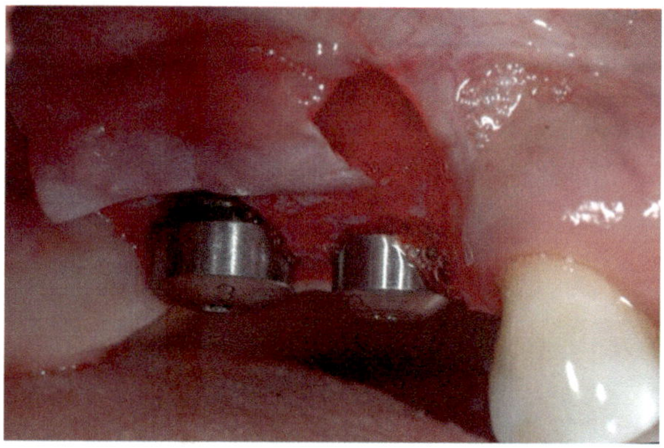

Fig. 4.29 Partial thickness flap

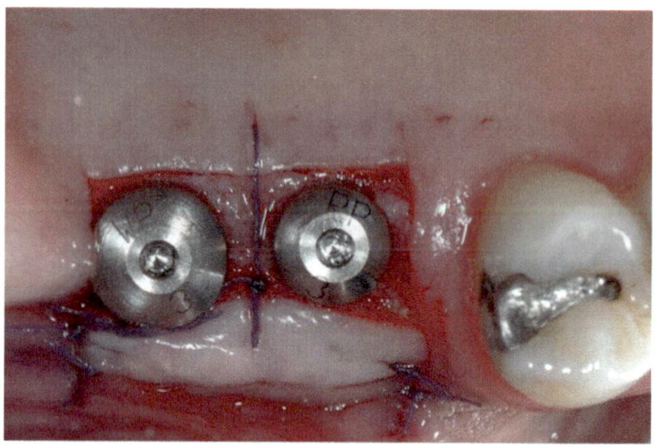

Fig. 4.30 Proper suturing technique

4.4.2 Free Gingival Graft

Free soft tissue graft can also be utilized to increase the zone of keratinized gingiva around dental implants. Due to the difference in color between the palatal donor site and the buccal recipient site, the esthetic outcomes may be compromised. In the following case, the author introduced a technique in which he used buccal keratinized gingiva as a donor site instead of the palatal site. Since harvesting tissues from the donor site can induce gingival recession around existing dentition, the dentist needs to make sure there is an abundance of tissues to harvest from without approaching the free gingival margin.

The following case is of a female patient who had immediate implant placement in the areas of tooth #5 with bone augmentation and resorbable collagen barrier (Figs. 4.31, 4.32, and 4.33). To achieve primary closure, the mucogingival junction

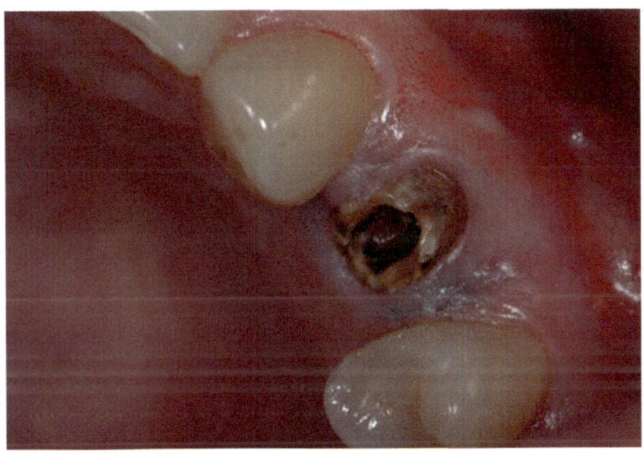

Fig. 4.31 Tooth #12 deemed hopeless

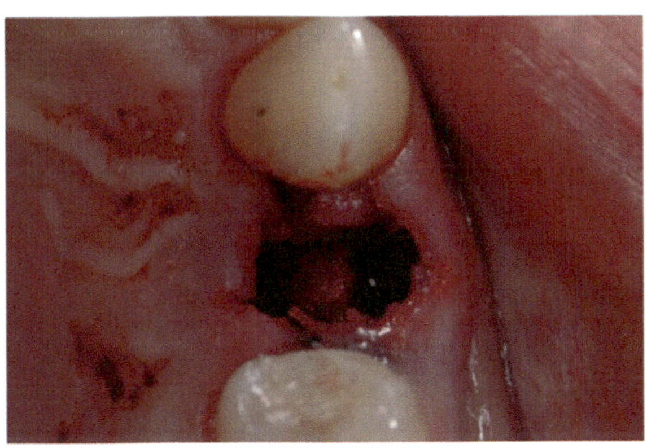

Fig. 4.32 Atraumatic extraction

was coronally displaced (Fig. 4.34). During the second stage, a free gingival graft was performed to compensate for the lack of keratinized gingiva on the buccal side of the implant (Fig. 4.35). The buccal side of teeth # 2–3 was used as a downer site

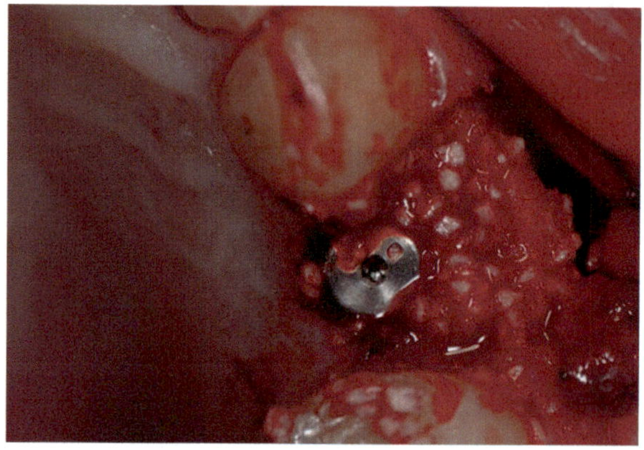

Fig. 4.33 Immediate placement with bone augmentation and GTR

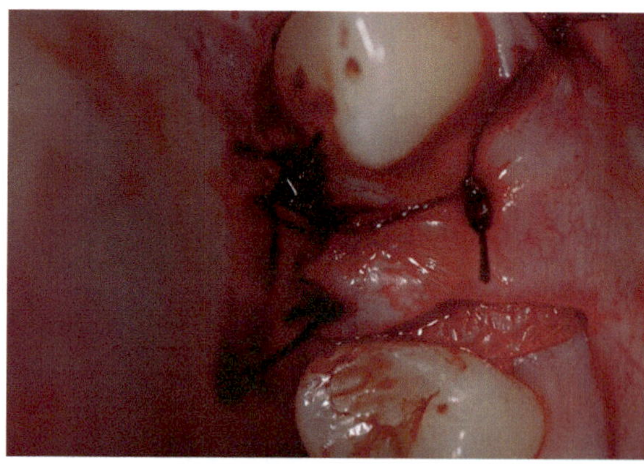

Fig. 4.34 Coronally displaced mucogingival junction

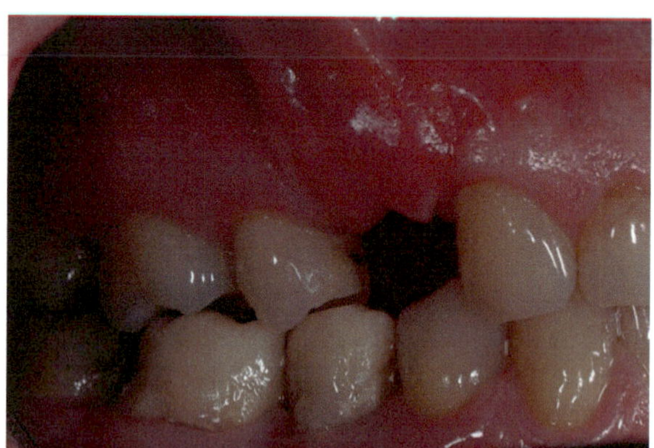

Fig. 4.35 Before the second stage

to harvest soft tissue graft, as shown in Figs. 4.36 and 4.37. Figure 4.38 shows the final implant-supported crown restoration.

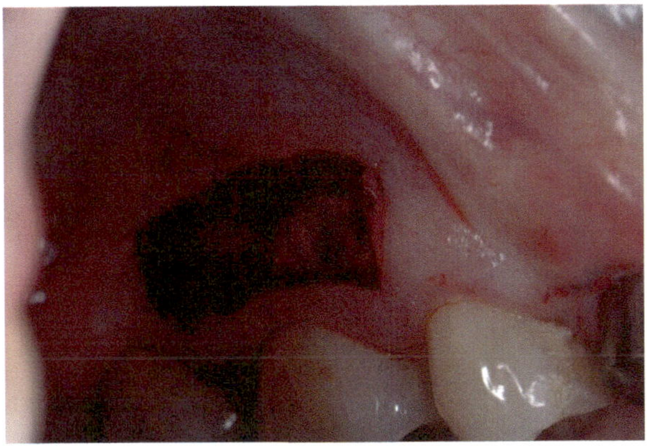

Fig. 4.36 Buccal downer site

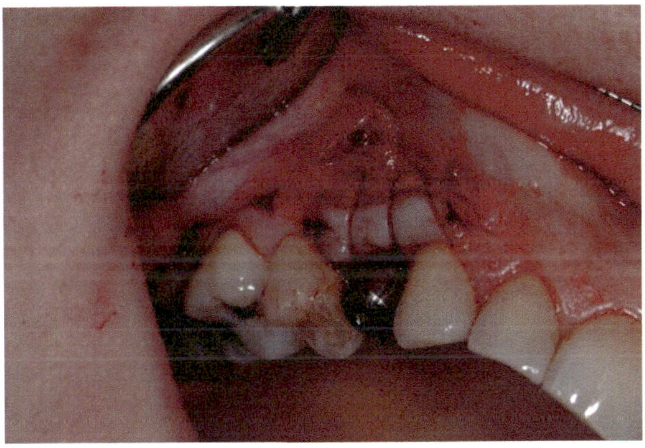

Fig. 4.37 FGG with healing abutment

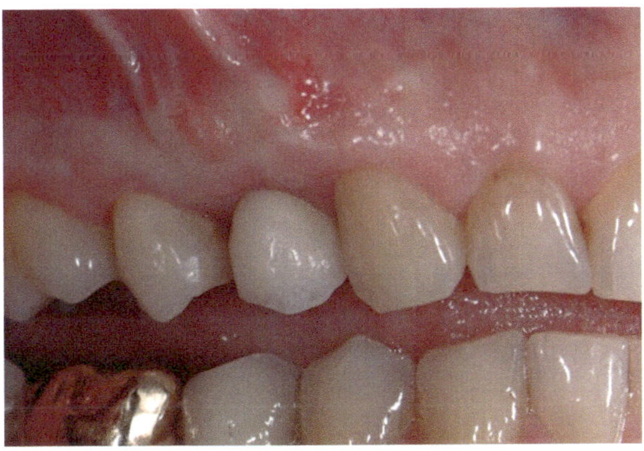

Fig. 4.38 Final implant-supported crown with FGG

4.4.3 Rotated Pedicle Flap

Since it was first published by Harvey, P.M in 1970, a pedicle flap has been implemented to manage and treat the lack of keratinized mucosa around dental apparatus. The next case shows how a rotated pedicle flap can be used while performing the second stage around implants to compensate for keratinized mucosa deficiency around implants (Figs. 4.39, 4.40, 4.41, 4.42, 4.43, and 4.44).

The following case is courtesy to Dr. Jose Nart.

4.4.4 Rotated Connective Tissue Graft

As a modification to the conventional connective tissue graft, this technique can be utilized to compensate for a lack of adequate thickness of soft tissue around dental implants.

Applying the same surgical principles of soft tissue grafting, the graft should be immobilized with adequate length and thickness and have enough vascularity to provide adequate blood supply to ensure graft survival. If the graft is meant to cover

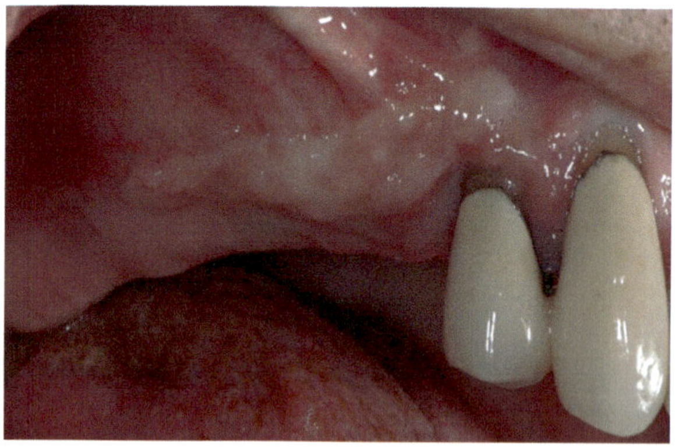

Fig. 4.39 Before performing the second stage

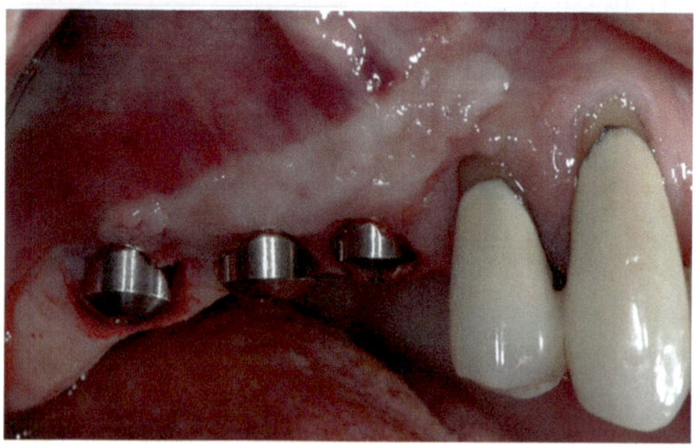

Fig. 4.40 Implant in the area of missing tooth #2 shows lack of keratinized mucosa

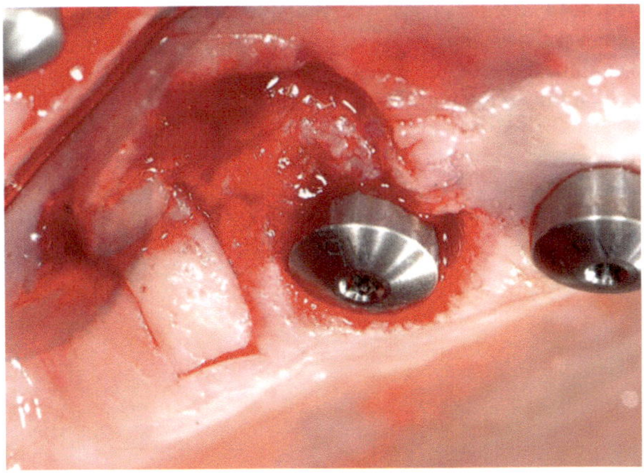

Fig. 4.41 Partial thickness flap before rotation

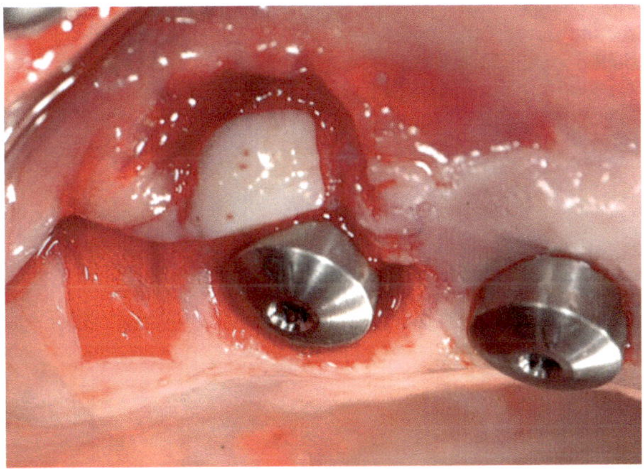

Fig. 4.42 Flap is placed passively on the buccal side of the implant

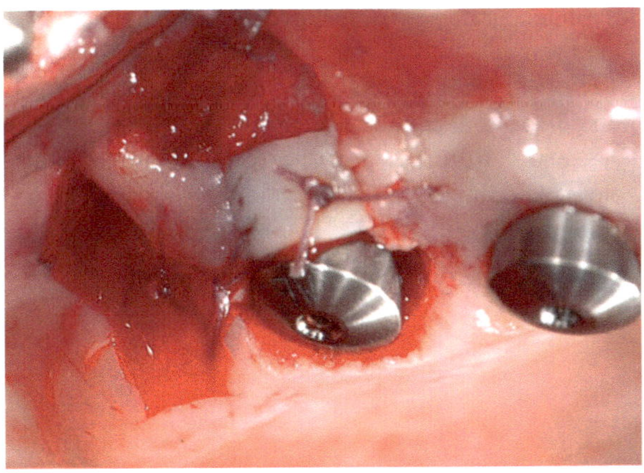

Fig. 4.43 Flap is sutured on buccal side

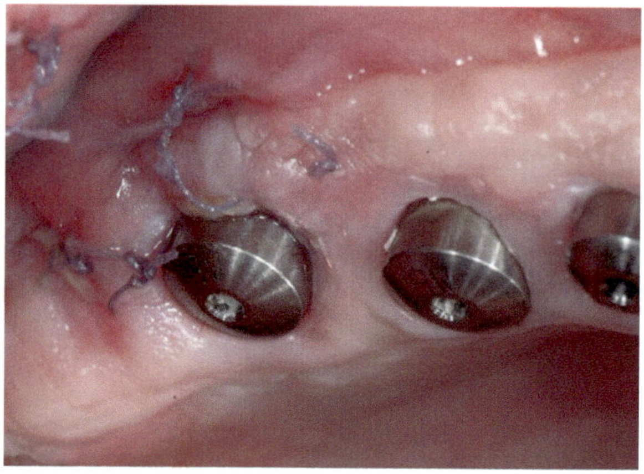

Fig. 4.44 Before suture removal shows more keratinized mucosa on the buccal side of the implant

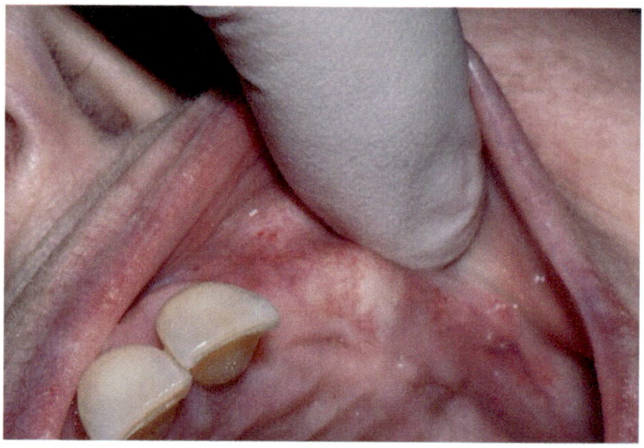

Fig. 4.45 Before the second stage of the implant on the maxillary left side

a surface that has no blood supply as in denuded roots or the implant surface, the practitioner must make sure there is enough blood supply coming from the peripheries of the graft by harvesting an adequately sized graft to provide the needed blood supply.

A newer technique has been introduced, which is called vascularized interpositional periosteal connective tissue flap (VIP-CT) [50]. Figs. 4.44, 4.45, 4.46, 4.47, 4.48, and 4.49 represent a case where that technique was utilized to increase the zona of keratinized tissues around four implants placed in the area of missing teeth of the maxillary left side. The procedure was completed during the second stage after allowing adequate time for osseointegration in preparation for the restorative phase.

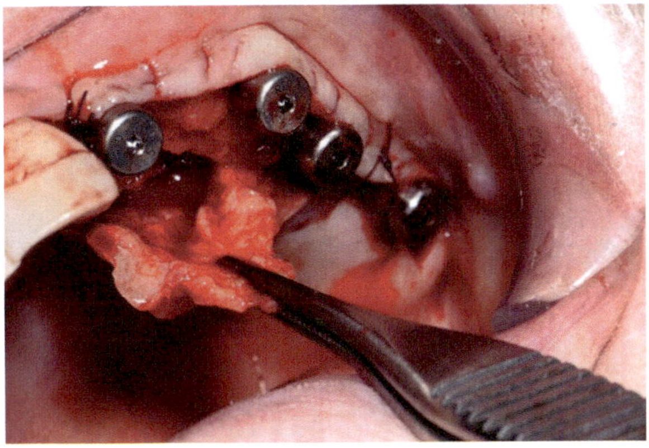

Fig. 4.46 VIP-CT around implants

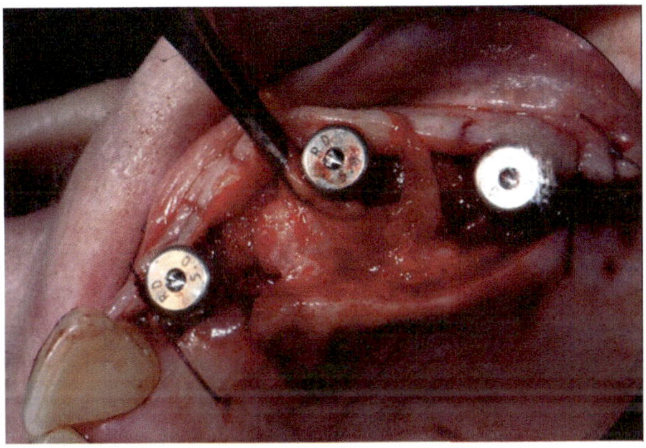

Fig. 4.47 Adapting the graft around the implant

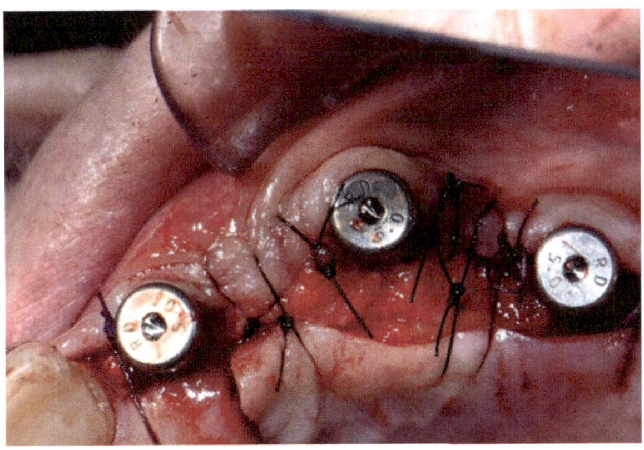

Fig. 4.48 Suturing while leaving the graft exposed

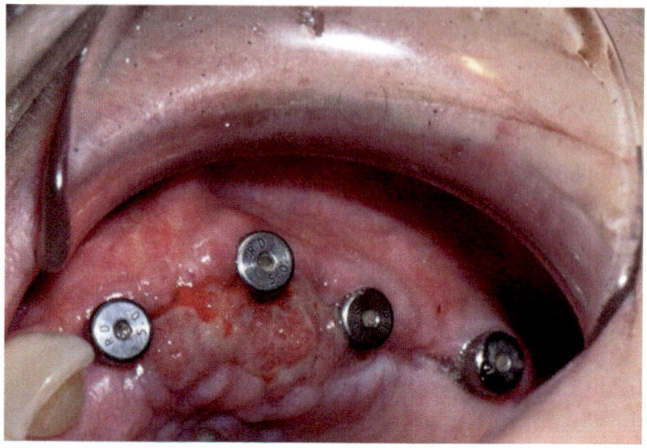

Fig. 4.49 Increased KT around the implant

4.5 After Loading

After implant loading and crown insertion, soft tissues around implants may exhibit some deficiencies. These deficiencies may lead to showing a black shadow of the implant body under a thin biotype or may result in gingival recessions. Thin tissues are prone to more recession, are susceptible to attachment loss and gingival displacement over time [51], and lack bone stabilization [52, 53].

Recession is prevalent around natural teeth as well as implants. This prevalence seems to be age related. For patients in their twenties, the rate of recession is about 27.9% [54] and increases to reach up to 100% of the population in their fifties [55]. Gingival recession may be related to traumatic injuries, such as faulty tooth brushing, which primarily affects the buccal surface of the maxillary anterior and premolar dentition [56]. Gingival recession may also result from an inflammatory reaction to bacteria-related plaque accumulation, which may occur around any tooth in the oral cavity [57].

Treating recession, whether around natural dentition or implants, is not guaranteed to result in complete coverage for the exposed portion of the root or implant fixture. As mentioned before, different gingival grafting techniques have been considered and applied in an attempt to achieve satisfactory results. The stability of soft tissues around implant-supported crowns is essential for long-term optimal aesthetic outcomes [58]. If recession is left untreated, it will affect the esthetic appearance, often negatively reflected in a patient's self-esteem [59]. Not only will grafting improve aesthetic results, but it will also augment the peri-implant gingival tissues in a way to allow patients to perform proper oral hygiene measures without pain and discomfort.

As defined by the glossary of periodontal terms (3rd edition, American Academy of Periodontology, 1992), recession is the location of the marginal periodontal tissues apical to the cemento-enamel junction. Given the morphological differences between periodontal and peri-implant tissues [60] and the related anatomical characteristics, it is reasonable to assume that a grafting procedure is more sophisticated around dental implants than natural dentitions. Caution should be practiced during surgical implant placement regarding hard bony structures [61]. A severe buccally positioned implant may lead to hard tissue dehiscence, which may negatively influence the peri-implant soft tissue position, leading to gingival recessions [62].

Approximately 24% of immediately placed implants will manifest gingival recession in 1-year follow-up [61]. The next section will discuss the two most commonly used techniques to correct soft tissue dificiencies around implants.

4.5.1 Autogenous Tissues

The surgeon can either harvest connective tissue or free epithelized gingival tissue grafts (FEGTG). The next section will focus on connective tissue grafts.

4.5.1.1 Connective Tissue Graft

Accompanied by a coronally positioned flap, the connective tissue graft is considered to be the gold standard technique of gingival tissue augmentation around natural teeth and implants [63], resulting in about 66% coverage at the 6-month follow-up [64]. Figures 4.50, 4.51, 4.52, and 4.53 show the restoration of a second mandibular premolar implant with a well-fitted crown. Two years later, the buccal side shows that the metal margin of the crown has become exposed due to gingival recession and a lack of adequate soft tissues. In an attempt to increase the zone of healthy thick gingiva and attain metal margin coverage, a gingival graft utilizing autogenous connective tissue was performed. The graft was completely covered under an envelope flap to ensure adequate blood supply. As shown in Fig. 4.54, the procedure resulted in a significant increase in the thickness and width of healthy gingival tissues, which will serve to improve esthetic as well as improve longevity.

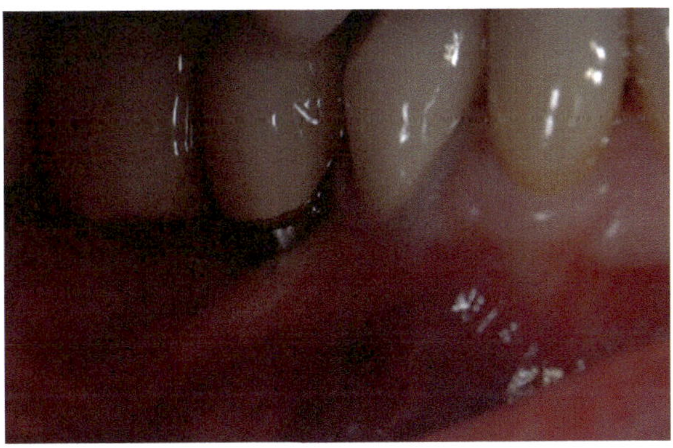

Fig. 4.50 Implant-supported crown with recession

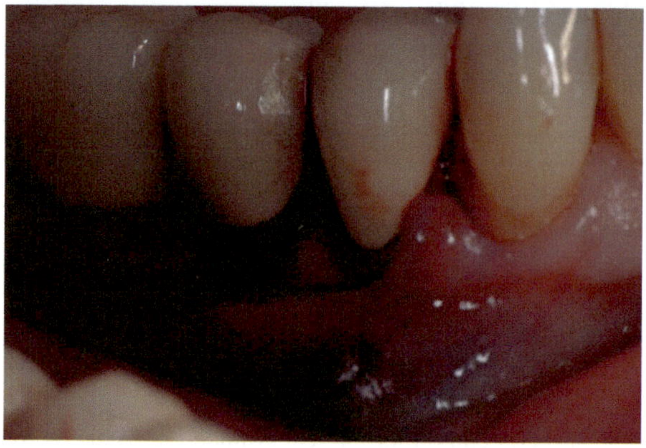

Fig. 4.51 Envelope flap with CTG

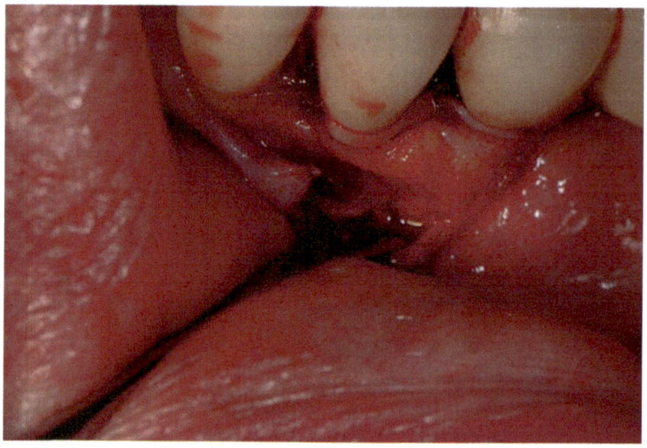

Fig. 4.52 CTG fixed on the implant's surface

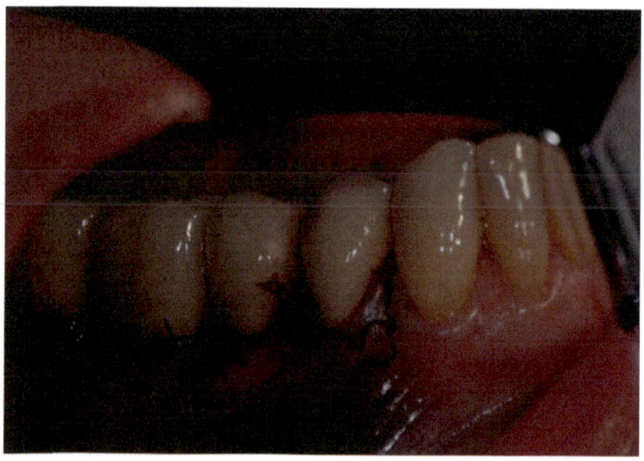

Fig. 4.53 Envelope flap sutured

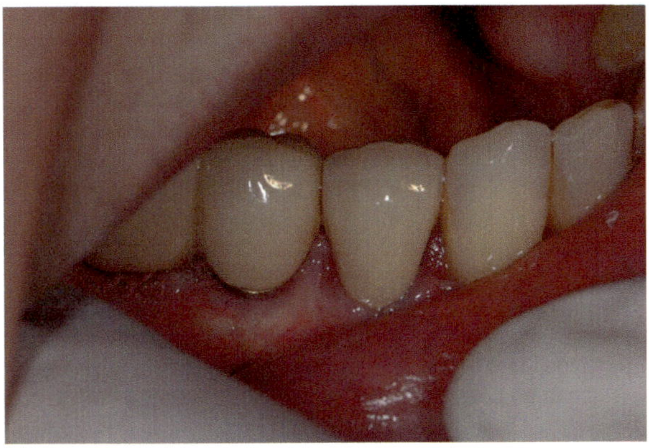

Fig. 4.54 6 weeks after graft with thicker biotype and some implant thread coverage

4.5.1.2 Free Gingival Graft

The same technique described before in Figs. 4.36, 4.37, and 4.38 can be utilized around restored implants.

4.5.2 Acellular Dermal Matrix Allograft (ADM)

This is a freeze-dried, cell-free, dermal matrix prepared by removing the epidermis and cellular components of human donor skin tissues [41]. The first documentation of the dental use of ADM was in 1996. It can act as a scaffold to allow repopulation of fibroblasts, blood vessels, and epithelium from surrounding tissues [65, 66]. ADM allows some advantages over the use of autogenous gingival tissue grafts: (1) it does not require additional wound of the donor site, (2) it avoids the limitation of autogenous tissues, and (3) Wie PC et al. reported better esthetic outcomes compared to autogenous tissues.

References

1. Buser D, Janner SF, Wittneben JG, Brägger U, Ramseier CA, Salvi GE. 10-year survival and success rates of 511 titanium implants with a sandblasted and acid-etched surface: a retrospective study in 303 partially edentulous patients. Clin Implant Dent Relat Res. 2012;14(6):839–51.
2. Iacono VJ, Committee on Research, Science and Therapy, The American Academy of Periodontology. Dental implants in periodontal therapy. J Periodontol. 2000;71:1934–42.
3. Bouri A Jr, Bissada N, Al-Zahrani MS, Faddoul F, Nouneh I. Width of keratinized gingiva and the health status of the supporting tissues around dental implants. Int J Oral Maxillofac Implants. 2008;23(2):1.
4. Yu-Wen C, Leebc S-Y, Linab Y-C, Lai Y-L. J Chin Med Assoc. 2015;78(7):389–94.

5. Bengazi F, Botticelli D, Favero V, Perini A, Urbizo Velez J, Lang NP. Influence of presence or absence of keratinized mucosa on the alveolar bony crest level as it relates to different buccal marginal bone thicknesses. An experimental study in dogs. Clin Oral Implants Res. 2014;25(9):1065–71. https://doi.org/10.1111/clr.12233; Epub 2013 Jul 29.
6. Oh SL, Masri RM, Williams DA, Ji C, Romberg E. Free gingival grafts for implants exhibiting lack of keratinized mucosa: a prospective controlled randomized clinical study. J Clin Periodontol. 2017;44(2):195–203. https://doi.org/10.1111/jcpe.12660.
7. Warrer K, Buser D, Lang NP, Karring T. Plaque-induced peri-implantitis in the presence or absence of keratinized mucosa. An experimental study in monkeys. Clin Oral Implants Res. 1995;6:131–8.
8. Boynuegri D, Nemli SK, Kasko YA. Significance of keratinized mucosa around dental implants: a prospective comparative study. Clin Oral Implants Res. 2013;24:928–33.
9. Zigdon H, Machtei EE. The dimensions of keratinized mucosa around implants affect clinical and immunological parameters. Clin Oral Implants Res. 2008;19:387–92.
10. Nabers CL. Repositioning the attached gingiva. J Periodontol. 1954;25:38–9.
11. Ochsenbein C. Newer concept of mucogingival surgery. J Periodontol. 1960;31:175–85.
12. Friedman L, Levine HL. Mucogingival surgery: current status. J Periodontol. 1964;35:5–21.
13. Carranza FA, Carraro JJ. Mucogingival techniques in periodontal surgery. J Periodontol. 1970;41:294–9.
14. Lang NP, Loe H. The relationship between the width of keratinized gingiva and gingival health. J Periodontol. 1972;43:623–7.
15. Miyasato M, Crigger M, Egelberg J. Gingival condition in areas of minimal and appreciable width of keratinized gingiva. J Clin Periodontol. 1977;4:200–9.
16. Wennstrom JL, Lindhe J. Plaque-induced gingival inflammation in the absence of attached gingiva in dogs. J Clin Periodontol. 1983;10:266–76.
17. Bassetti M, Kaufmann R, Salvi GE, et al. Soft tissue grafting to improve the attached mucosa at dental implants: a review of the literature and proposal of a decision tree. Quintessence Int. 2015;46:499–510.
18. Berglundh T, Lindhe J, Jonsson K, et al. The topography of the vascular systems in the periodontal and peri-implant tissues in the dog. J Clin Periodontol. 1994;21:189–93.
19. Berglundh T, Lindhe J, Ericsson I, et al. The soft tissue barrier at implants and teeth. Clin Oral Implants Res. 1991;2:81–90.
20. Listgarten MA, Lang NP, Schroeder HE, et al. Periodontal tissues and their counterparts around endosseous implants [corrected and republished with original paging, article orginally printed in Clin Oral Implants Res 1991 Jan-mar;2(1):1-19]. Clin Oral Implants Res. 1991;2:1–19.
21. Zangrando MS, Damante CA, Sant'Ana AC, Rubo de Rezende ML, Greghi SL, Chambrone L. Long-term evaluation of periodontal parameters and implant outcomes in periodontally compromised patients: a systematic review. J Periodontol. 2015;86:201–21.
22. Wennstrom JL, Derks J. Is there a need for keratinized mucosa around implants to maintain health and tissue stability. Clin Oral Implants Res. 2012;23(Suppl):136–46.
23. Roccuzzo M, De Angelis N, Bonino L, Bunino M, Bonino F. Keratinized mucosa and soft tissues conditions around posterior mandibular implants. (French) Journal de Parodontologie & d'Implantologie Orale. 2010;29:261–7.
24. Souza AB, Tormena M, Matarazzo F, et al. The influence of peri-implant keratinized mucosa on brushing discomfort and peri-implant tissue health. Clin Oral Implants Res. 2015;27(6):650–5.
25. Bassetti RG, Stähli A, Bassetti MA, Sculean A. Soft tissue augmentation around osseointegrated and uncovered dental implants: a systematic review. Clin Oral Investig. 2017;21(1):53–70.
26. Puisys A, Linkevicius T. The influence of mucosal tissue thickening on crestal bone stability around bone-level implants. A prospective controlled clinical trial. Clin Oral Implants Res. 2015;26:123–9.
27. Linkevicius T, Puisys A, Linkeviciene L, et al. Crestal bone stability around implants with horizontally matching connection after soft tissue thickening: a prospective clinical trial. Clin Implant Dent Relat Res. 2015;17:497–508.

28. Buyukozdemir Askin S, Berker E, Akincibay H, et al. Necessity of keratinized tissues for dental implants: a clinical, immunological, and radiographic study. Clin Implant Dent Relat Res. 2015;17:1–12.
29. Costa FO, Takenaka-Martinez S, Cota LO, et al. Peri-implant disease in subjects with and without preventive maintenance: a 5-year follow-up. J Clin Periodontol. 2012;39:173–81.
30. Linkevicius T, Apse P, Grybauskas S, et al. The influence of soft tissue thickness on crestal bone changes around implants: a 1-year prospective controlled clinical trial. Int J Oral Maxillofac Implants. 2009;24:712–9.
31. Hürzeler MB, Weng D. Periimplant tissue management: optimal timing for an aesthetic result. Pract Periodontics Aesthet Dent. 1996;8:857–69; quiz 869.
32. Shibli JA, D'avila S, Marcantonio E Jr. Connective tissue graft to correct peri-implant soft tissue margin: a clinical report. J Prosthet Dent. 2004;91:119–22.
33. Yan JJ, Tsai AY, Wong MY, et al. Comparison of acellular dermal graft and palatal autograft in the reconstruction of keratinized gingiva around dental implants: a case report. Int J Periodontics Restorative Dent. 2006;26:287–92.
34. Chambrone L, Pannuti CM, Tu YK, Chambrone LA. Evidence-based periodontal plastic surgery. II. An individual data meta-analysis for evaluating factors in achieving complete root coverage. J Periodontal. 2012;83(4):477–90.
35. Gary HG, Longaker MT. Scarless wound healing. New York, NY: Dekker; 2000.
36. Sullivan HC, Atkins JH. Free autogenous gingival grafts. III. Utilization of grafts in the treatment of gingival recession. Periodontics. 1968;6:152–60.
37. Agudio G, Nieri M, Rotundo R, Cortellini P, Pini Prato G. Free gingival grafts to increase keratinized tissue: a retrospective long-term evaluation (10 to 25 years) of outcomes. J Periodontol. 2008;79:587–94.
38. Harvey PM. Surgical reconstruction of the gingiva. Part II. Procedure. N Z Dent J. 1970;66:42–54.
39. Griffin TJ, Cheung WS, Zavras AI, Damoulis PD. Postoperative complications following gingival augmentation procedures. J Periodontol. 2006;77:2070–9.
40. Wei PC, Laurrel L, Geivelis M, Lingen MW, Maddalozzo D. Acellular dermal matrix allografts to achieve increased attached gingiva. Part 1. Clinical study. J Periodontol. 2000;71:1297–305.
41. Rhee PH, Fiedman CD, Ridge A, Kusiak I. The use of processed allograft dermal matrix for intraoral resurfacing: an alternative to split-thickness skin grafts. Arch Otolaryngol Head Neck Surg. 1998;124:1201–4.
42. Kleinheinz J, Büchter A, Kruse-Lösler B, Weingart D, Joos U. Incision design in implant dentistry based on vascularization of the mucosa. Clin Oral Implants Res. 2005;16(5):518–23.
43. Kleinheinz J, Büchter A, Fillies T, Joos U. Vascular basis of mucosal color. Head Face Med. 2005;1:4.
44. Kinsel RP, Lamb RE. Development of gingival esthetics in the edentulous patient with immediately loaded, single stage, implant supported fixed prosthesis: a clinical report. Int J Oral Maxillofac Implants. 2000;15:711–21.
45. Esposito M, Murray-Curtis L, Grusovin MG, Coulthard P, Worthington HV. Interventions for replacing missing teeth: different types of dental implants. Cochrane Database Syst Rev. 2007;17:4.
46. Arisan V, Karabuda CZ, Ozdemir T. Implant surgery using bone- and mucosa-supported stereolithographic guides in totally edentulous jaws: surgical and post-operative outcomes of computer-aided vs. standard techniques. Clin Oral Implants Res. 2010;21:980–8.
47. Rocci A, Martignoni M, Gottlow J. Immediate loading in the maxilla using flapless surgery, implants placed in predetermined positions, and prefabricated provisional restorations: a restrospective 3-year clinical study. Clin Implant Dent Relat Res. 2003;5(suppl 1):29–36.
48. Sunitha RV, Sapthagiri E. Flapless implant surgery: a 2-year follow-up study of 40 implants. Oral Surg Oral Med Oral Pathol Oral Radiol. 2013;116:e237–43.
49. De Bruyn H, Atashkadeh M, Cosyn J, van de Velde T. Clinical outcome and bone preservation of single TiUnite™ implants installed with flapless or flap surgery. Clin Implant Dent Relat Res. 2011;13:175–83.

50. Chitra Agarwal, AB Tarun Kumar, MG Triveni, Dhoom Singh Mehta Vascularized interpositional periosteal connective tissues flap technique to correct soft tissue defect around maxillary anterior implant.
51. Serino G, Wennstro MJ, Lindhe J, Eneroth L. The prevalence and distribution of gingival recession in subjects with a high standard of oral hygiene. J Clin Periodontol. 1994;21:57–63.
52. Berglundh T, Lindhe J. Dimension of the periimplant mucosa. Biological width revisited. J Clin Periodontol. 1996;23:971–3.
53. Abrahamsson I, Berglundh T, Glantz PO, Lindhe J. The mucosal attachment at different abutments. An experimental study in dogs. J Clin Periodontol. 1998;25:721–7.
54. Raetzke R. Parodontale Rezessionen–Pra¨valenz, Signifikanz, Ursachen und Therapie. Zahna¨rztliche Wissenschaftliche Revue. 1985;94:968–74.
55. Loe H, Anerud A, Boysen H. The natural history of periodontal disease in man: prevalence, severity and extent of gingival recession. J Periodontol. 1992;63:489–95.
56. Sangnes G, Gjermo P. Prevalence of soft and hard tissue lesions related to mechanical tooth cleaning procedures. Community Dent Oral Epidemiol. 1976;4:77–83.
57. Baelum V, Fejerskov O, Karring T. Oral hygiene, gingivitis and periodontal breakdown in adult Tanzanians. J Periodontal Res. 1986;21:221–32.
58. Belser UC, Buser D, Hess D, Schmid B, Bernard JP, Lang NP. Esthetic implant restorations in partially edentulous patients—a critical appraisal. Periodontology 2000. 1998;17:132–50.
59. Burkhardt R, Andreoni C, Marinello C. Psychological and social effects of implant-supported reconstructions. Acta Med Dentium Helvetica. 2000;5:1–8.
60. Listgarten MA, Lang NP, Schroeder HE, Schroeder A. Periodontal tissues and their counterparts around endosseous implants. Clin Oral Implants Res. 1991;2:1–19.
61. Cosyn J, Sabzevar MM, De Bruyn H. Predictors of interproximal and midfacial recession following single implant treatment in the anterior maxilla: a multivariate analysis. J Clin Periodontol. 2012;39:895–903.
62. Benic GI, Mokti M, Chen CJ, Weber HP, Hammerle CH, Gallucci GO. Dimensions of buccal bone and mucosa at immediately placed implants after 7 years: a clinical and cone beam computed tomography study. Clin Oral Implants Res. 2012;23:560–6.
63. Chambrone L, Tatakis DN. Periodontal soft tissue root coverage procedures: a systematic review from the AAP regeneration workshop. J Periodontol. 2015;86:S8–51.
64. Burkhardt R, Joss A, Lang NP. Soft tissue dehiscence coverage around endosseous implants: a prospective cohort study. Clin Oral Implants Res. 2008;19:451–7.
65. Wei PC, Laurell L, Lingen MW, et al. Acellular dermal matrix allografts to achieve increased attached gingiva. Part 2. A histological comparative study. J Periodontol. 2002;73:1299–130.
66. Gapski R, Park CA, Wang HL. Acellular dermal matrix for mucogingival surgery: a meta analysis. J Periodontol. 2005;76:1814–22.

5 Proper Oral Hygiene Measures to Maintain Healthy Soft Tissues Around Dental Implants

Irene Kim, Kevin Lin, and Soo Woo Kim

5.1 Introduction

With the advancement in dentistry, the placement of dental implants has become a routine procedure for the rehabilitation of fully and partially edentulous patients. However, with the increasing number of implants, there is an increasing number of cases with peri-implant diseases. As there are no established and predictable concepts for the treatment of peri-implantitis, primary prevention—the management of peri-implant mucositis to prevent the onset of peri-implantitis—is of key importance before the consequences become irreversible [1].

5.2 Peri-Implant Health and Disease: Epidemiology

Despite the high survival rate of implants, peri-implant disease, such as peri-implant mucositis, and peri-implantitis, can occur in some cases. Peri-implant mucositis is defined as the development of mucosal inflammation around the implant without any loss of supporting bone. Peri-implantitis is defined by the inflammatory process of the soft and hard tissue around the imp lant that leads to peri-implant pocket formation with loss of supporting bone. It is often associated with increased probing depths with bleeding on probing and/or suppuration and mucosal recession. There are many studies that discuss a wide range of prevalence of peri-implantitis and

I. Kim
Private Practice, New York, NY, USA

K. Lin
Private Practice, San Diego, CA, USA

S. W. Kim (✉)
Department of Oral Medicine, Infection and Immunity, Harvard School of Dental Medicine, Boston, MA, USA
e-mail: Soo-woo_kim@hsdm.harvard.edu

M. Hassan (ed.), *Peri-Implant Soft Tissue Management*,
https://doi.org/10.1007/978-3-031-45516-2_5

peri-implant mucositis. A meta-analysis estimated a weighted mean prevalence of 43% for peri-implant mucositis and 22% for peri-implantitis [2–4].

Plaque-induced peri-implantitis is one of the most common complications. Therefore, to prevent further breakdown and inflammatory processes around the peri-implant, oral hygiene and nonsurgical measures are essential.

5.3 Importance of Oral Hygiene

In a retrospective study, Costa et al. discussed that the lack of annual supportive therapy in patients diagnosed with peri-implant mucositis showed an increased risk of developing peri-implantitis. In a group of subjects that did not receive annual maintenance, 43.9% presented with peri-implantitis, whereas the subjects who complied with supportive therapy presented with 18% of peri-implantitis [5].

Literature shows that plaque control is a critical aspect in maintaining peri-implant health and preventing the future progression to peri-implant mucositis and peri-implantitis.

5.4 Dental Implant Design

Similar to the gingival tissue at teeth, the peri-implant mucosa forms a junctional epithelium that faces the titanium surface. The collagen fibers appear to commence at the marginal bone and remain parallel with the abutment surface. However, the gingival attachment to the implants is weaker than that of natural teeth as there is no connective tissue attachment, which makes it susceptible to inflammation [6].

In addition, reduced vasculature around the implant compared to the natural tooth makes detection of inflammation more difficult. Bleeding of probing is one of the key risk indicators for peri-implant mucositis, but it shouldn't be the sole indicator since reduced vasculature lowers the sensitivity of detection. Therefore, close monitoring of the provider around the implant is essential for early detection of peri-implant mucositis [7–9].

Subgingival plaque removal around implants is difficult due to the implant design and placement of the implants. Usually, in an esthetically-demanding anterior region, the implants are often placed subgingivally and, in some cases, below the alveolar crest to create an adequate emergence profile. These factors should be considered at the stage of planning implant treatment for better maintenance of peri-implant health [10].

The clinical success of dental implants is dependent on the osseointegration of the implant through the direct contact between bone and the implant. Thus, various surface characteristics of dental implants are available, ranging from relatively smooth machine surfaces to a more roughened surface. The roughened surfaces accelerate healing and promote osseointegration, achieved through modifications of the surface topography by mechanical, chemical, electrochemical, and laser treatments [11, 12].

With the ongoing modifications, there has been an increased focus on peri-implant health, the incidence of bone loss, and whether the different surface roughness has an effect. Based on comparative studies, it can be concluded that the average peri-implant bone loss around the moderately rough and minimally rough surface was less than that of rough surface implants [13].

The modified surfaces challenge providers and patients for proper maintenance around the implant once exposed outside of bone and gingiva. Due to the surface topology, it will retain more bacteria and make complete removal nearly impossible. Prevention of exposure to surface outside bone/gingiva is essential for the long-term maintenance of the implant, which should be considered even in the planning of implant treatment [14, 15].

5.5 Provider vs. Patients

The effective management of peri-implant mucositis requires patient-administered measures in conjunction with professional-administered plaque removal procedures.

Professionally administered plaque removal procedures include oral hygiene instructions, air abrasive devices, polishing tools, and mechanical debridement with the use of a variety of hand or powered instruments. These measures showed a reduction in clinical signs of inflammation. Salvi et al. showed a significant improvement and reverse of peri-implant mucositis with the use of professionally administered plaque removal and reinforcement of oral hygiene instructions [16].

Patient-administered measures include manual or powered toothbrushes for mechanical plaque removal and triclosan-containing toothpaste and adjunctive antimicrobials for chemical plaque control. In the studies in the meta-analysis by Salvi et al., the complete resolution of inflammation, the absence of bleeding on probing, was not always reported; however, a reduction of clinical signs of inflammation was evident. Thus, the need for professionally administered plaque removal is justified [17, 18].

5.5.1 Provider's Care

The intervals for professionally administered supportive care should be established according to the individual's periodontal status and self-care. Recommended recall interval should be 5 to 6 months [2, 19, 20]. During these recall visits, peri-implant tissues must be regularly examined to monitor any changes for the early detection, prevention, and treatment of peri-implant disease [9].

During the recall exam, the dental professional should question the patient about any pain or concerns. The clinical exam will be followed by assessments of the dental implants for the presence of plaque and calculus accumulation, examining for signs of inflammation and peri-implant soft tissue color and consistency and probing depths, including bleeding on probing. A radiographic analysis can be done to determine bone loss [9, 14, 21, 22].

5.5.1.1 Radiographs

Alberektsson et al. discussed the criteria for the success of dental implants, which includes bone loss of less than 0.2 mm annually after the implant's first year of service [23]. Thus, an essential pre- and post-operative tool to evaluate the success of the implant is the use of radiographs. Radiograph images can be used to evaluate the change in bone height overtime. It is recommended to take a radiograph for baseline after implant placement, after the insertion of the prosthesis, and during maintenance care as needed [12, 24]. A periapical or vertical bitewing radiograph can be taken at 6 to 8 months and 1 year to compare to the baseline. When no change in the crestal bone level is evident, subsequent radiographs can be taken every 3 years. However, if unfavorable clinical signs and crestal changes are observed, it is recommended to take additional radiographs every 6 to 8 months until the bone level is stable for two consecutive periods [25]. The interface between the implant and the bone level should be well delineated.

5.5.1.2 Probing Depths

When probing, either a metal or plastic probe can be used. Studies showed that the gentle insertion of either a metal or plastic probe did not interfere or damage the mucosal attachment around the implant. However, a plastic probe may reduce the potential trauma to the peri-mucosal seal. In addition, many clinicians advocate the use of a flexible plastic probe as it is helpful when navigating around the height of contour of a dental implant prosthesis [14].

It is important to note the difference between the soft tissue around the implant and a natural tooth. Dental implants have a weaker hemidesmosomal attachment and are more fragile compared to a natural tooth. This makes probing around the implants more sensitive than teeth, and thus more gentle insertion of the probe is necessary [26, 27].

When probing the implants, the depth of the probing depth is not as meaningful as it is with the natural teeth, as the implant may have been placed deeper and the sulcus was created surgically. Therefore, it is essential to note whether there is bleeding on probing around implants as it is thought to be a predictor for peri-implantitis. Lang et al. demonstrated that healthy peri-implant sites were characterized by the absence of bleeding, whereas peri-implant mucositis and peri-implantitis showed increased bleeding on probing. Thus, the conjunction of measuring the probing depths and bleeding on probing can be used to monitor the condition of the peri-implant soft tissues [28].

5.5.1.3 Presence of Plaque/Calculus

The clinician should evaluate and record the presence of plaque and calculus accumulation around the dental implant. This can be done with or without the use of disclosing tablets. This allows for a longitudinal assessment of the patient's oral hygiene and compliance. At this visit, the review and reinforcement of oral hygiene is essential.

5.5.1.4 Signs of Inflammation

The presence of purulent exudates has been associated with peri-implantitis. Suppuration is a definite indicator of disease activity and, when noted, should take measures for anti-infective therapy immediately.

5.5.1.5 Instruments

Once the peri-implant status and the condition of the implant prosthesis are evaluated, plaque control is done for implant maintenance. Professional hygiene care combines the use of powered and manual devices in the debridement of the implant surface and abutment. It includes scaling and curettage using plastic instruments, titanium scalers, gold-plated curettes, and ultrasonic or sonic scalers with plastic-covered and novel metallic copper alloy tips. This is followed by polishing with the use of a rubber cup with polishing paste that is nonabrasive or air-powder polishing [9].

The instruments should be effective in removing plaque without damaging the implant surfaces. The use of metallic instruments or vigorous scaling can scratch the implant surface and result in alterations that make it susceptible to bacterial plaque and calculus accumulation and inflammation of the soft tissue. Thus, gentle debridement is recommended [24]. Many studies compare the use of different instruments for implant maintenance and how they affect the implant surfaces. The use of metal curettes and ultrasonic instruments reported severe roughness, scarring, and pitting of the titanium and hydroxyapatite-coated surfaces. On the other hand, plastic scalers maintained the integrity of the implant surfaces. In a comparative study, there was no significant difference in the titanium implant surface following the use of titanium, stainless steel, or plastic curettes, whereas the metal instruments caused surface alterations [29].

5.5.1.6 Scaling

The use of plastic instruments is advocated to decrease the possibility of scratching the implant surface as it produces insignificant alterations [30]. Upon insertion of the instrument, the blade should be against the implant abutment, engaging past the deposit apically with the stroke extending coronally. Horizontal, oblique, vertical short, and light-pressured strokes should be used to prevent trauma of the peri-implant tissue [24].

In some instances where the prosthesis limits access and prevents the insertion of the hand instruments, ultrasonic scalers can be used (Fig. 5.1). As ultrasonics can cause damage to the surface, newly developed plastic-covered and novel metallic copper alloy ultrasonic scaler tips (Fig. 5.2) [31] can be used to remove deposits. Recent findings showed that these tips showed minimal negative effects on the titanium surface [14].

5.5.1.7 Polishing

The use of a rubber cup with a nonabrasive polishing paste, such as aluminum oxide, tin oxide, and APF-free prophy paste, produced minimal surface alterations on the implant titanium surface. In instances where a polishing paste is not used, an antibacterial solution such as chlorhexidine can be used.

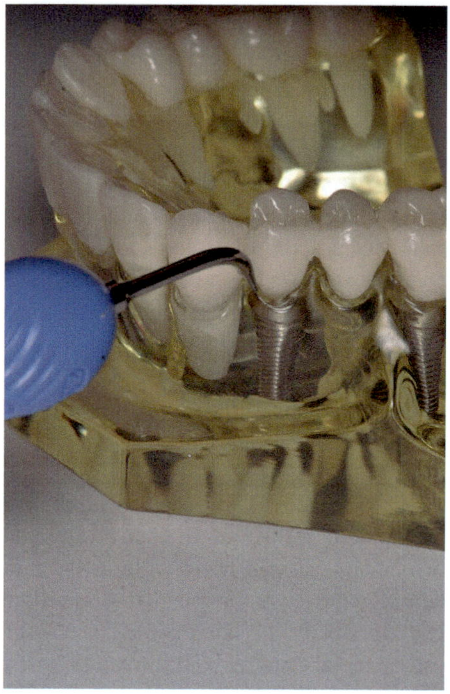

Fig. 5.1 A proper technique to hold ultra-sonic scaler around the implant. The tip must be parallel to the implant crown. It should not be touching the implant/abutment surface

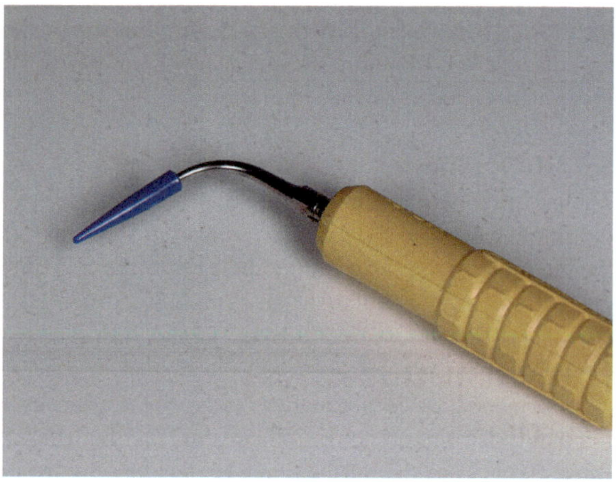

Fig. 5.2 A plastic-covered novel metallic copper alloy ultrasonic scaler tip. The blue plastic cover is replaceable

The use of air polishing devices is a controversial topic when it comes to dental implants. Literature shows conflicting reports on the efficacy of air polishing. Some studies indicate that air polishing is safe and effective in removing plaque compared to a curette. It effectively removes microorganisms and allows the normal fibroblast growth in vitro. However, others have reported that airbrushing can cause damage to the porcelain and composite material, create pitting and surface irregularities on the titanium surface, and leave powder deposits on the surface. The air pressure may also interfere with the peri-mucosal seal by detaching the soft tissue connection from the implant [24, 32].

Studies compared the use of glycine powder and sodium bicarbonate ($NaHCO_3$) powder. As sodium bicarbonate was shown to be abrasive, amino-acid glycine salt was introduced to minimize the trauma to the soft tissue. The mean size of the glycine powder particle is less than 45 μm with a maximum particle size of 60 μm, whereas the sodium bicarbonate particle size is four times larger [33]. Therefore, various studies demonstrated that the use of glycine powder was less abrasive and more efficient in the removal of the subgingival biofilm compared with sodium bicarbonate powder [34].

Despite the emphasis on the use of instruments or devices that do not cause alterations to the implant titanium surfaces, no studies have yet linked the scratching of the implant surface to increased incidences of peri-mucositis or peri-implantitis [14, 35].

5.5.2 Patient's Care

5.5.2.1 Home Care for Patients

Proper maintenance of dental implants is crucial for long-term success of dental implant therapy. As with natural teeth, inflammation resulting from biofilm accumulation around a dental implant is an etiologic factor for peri-implant mucositis and peri-implantitis. While professional maintenance during routine recall appointments is important, motivating and educating the patients on the proper home care regimen is paramount. Due to the anatomical differences between a natural tooth and an implant restoration, many of the same oral hygiene products and techniques easily translate to or are easily adapted for use around dental implants [36–38].

5.5.2.2 Manual Toothbrush Technique

There is a wide range in the design of manual toothbrushes, but there is limited research evidence to show whether one design is better than another. The consensus is that a soft bristle toothbrush is as effective as a hard bristle toothbrush with less risk of unnecessary trauma to the soft and hard tissues [39].

Brushing technique should not be different for natural dentitions and dentitions with implants. There are four main hand-brushing techniques that will be described below.

Bass (Sulcular) Technique

Charles Cassidy Bass described the Bass technique in 1948, advocating the use of the Right Kind brush with an intrasulcular technique. The toothbrush is placed parallel to the teeth, with the bristles pointing toward the gingiva. The brush is tilted 45 degrees, and the bristles are moved slightly subgingivally (Fig. 5.3). Gentle pressure and back-and-forth strokes are used while maintaining the subgingival position of the bristles. The lingual surfaces of the teeth are cleaned in a similar manner.

Depending on the location and angulation of the implant, 45-degree angle could be adjusted to reach the sulcus area [40].

Modified Bass Technique

The Modified Bass Technique is a modification by Columbia University of the original Bass technique. In this technique, the head of the toothbrush is held at 45 degrees against the teeth with bristles on both the tooth and gingiva. This allows the bristles to reach subgingivally. The toothbrush is moved in a circular motion to gently slide the bristles under the gingiva and remove plaque. The modification made by Columbia was to improve the removal of plaque from the gingival crevice. To do this, the brush is rolled from the gingival margin toward the occlusal surface of the teeth. This motion is repeated for the buccal and lingual surfaces of the teeth [40].

Stationary Bristle Technique

The Stationary Bristle Technique is another modification of the original Bass Technique. The goal of this technique is to avoid the scrubbing motion, which can lead to abrasion, gingival recession, and trauma. Like the Bass Technique, the bristles are aimed cervically into the gingival crevice. With very short vibratory strokes, care is taken to activate the bristle tips without bristle tip movement [41].

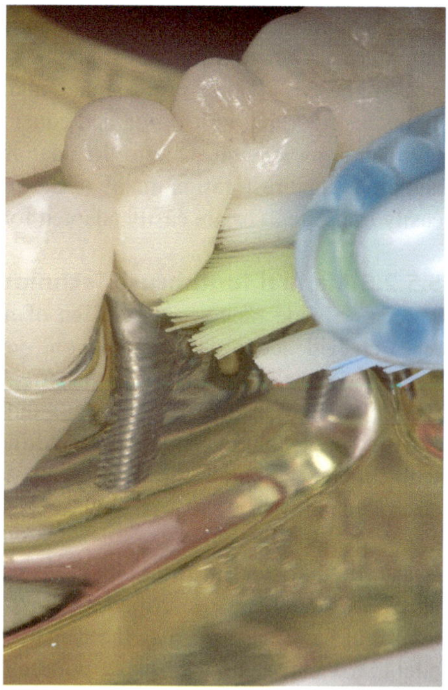

Fig. 5.3 Bass technique. The bristle of the brush should be tilted 45 degrees and inserted into the crevice of gingival margin

Stillman's Technique

The Stillman's technique is not an intrasulcular technique. Rather, the toothbrush bristles are placed on the gingiva and swept toward the occlusal surface of teeth with a rolling and vibratory motion. This technique may help to remove more interproximal plaque and also avoid gingival trauma in the case of thin gingival biotype or post-operatively after gingival surgery. This technique might not be sufficient to maintain proper hygiene around the implant [42].

5.5.2.3 Power Toothbrush Technique

There are currently many manufacturers of power toothbrushes, but the two largest players are Sonicare and Oral-B. The Sonicare toothbrush oscillates at a frequency of 31,000 strokes per second while the Oral-B toothbrush vibrates at 31,000 strokes per minute, rotates between 7600 and 8800 rotations/oscillations per minute, and pulses from 20,000 to 30,000 pulses per minute. The efficacy of the two electric toothbrushes is similar. These oscillations and strokes help make power toothbrushes very efficient at plaque removal, but patients still need to focus on proper brushing techniques [43–45]. Because the power toothbrush provides most of the cleaning power, there is no need for the patient to "scrub" their teeth and the patient can focus on angling the bristles properly into the gingival crevice like the Stationary Bristle Technique and moving slowly the bristles onto the tooth by tooth instead of moving toothbrush back and forth [46–51].

5.5.2.4 Interproximal Cleaning

Dental Floss/Tape/Superfloss

The most common and traditional way to clean interproximally between teeth is with dental floss. While there is a wide variety of floss on the market, it is advisable to use unwaxed tape or any floss that does not shred or leave behind particles in the gingival sulcus. Floss can be used with the same technique with single implants and teeth. However, for implant-supported fixed prostheses or bar-retained prostheses, a floss threader may be needed in order to thread the floss under the prosthesis. Alternatively, superfloss, which contains a threader, a wide band of ribbon, and normal floss, all in one product, can be very effective in removing plaque around implants. The threader portion can be introduced from buccal to lingual interproximally and wrapped around the tooth and reintroduced from lingual to buccal interproximally. The ends of the superfloss are criss-crossed on the buccal side, and the ribbon portion is used in a "shoe-shine" motion to circumferentially clean the implant surface (Fig. 5.4). This is particularly effective because of the narrow and circular shape of the implant body [52].

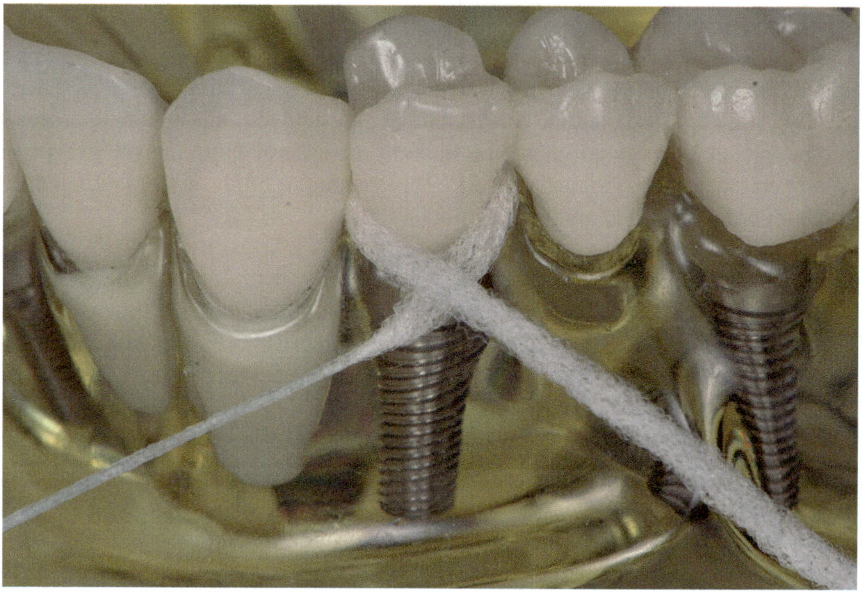

Fig. 5.4 A "shoe-shine" motion of the superfloss. This motion will circumferentially clean the implant surface

Interproximal Brush

For patients with limited dexterity, interproximal brushes offer an effective way to clean interproximally. Care must be taken to use a nylon-coated interproximal brush. There are brushes on the market with a metal wire that can potentially scratch and damage the implant surface. Additionally, some manufacturers offer interproximal brushes in multiple sizes and shapes. The particular brush should be chosen based on the manufacturer's recommendations. To use, the interproximal brush is inserted interdentally while applying a circular motion to effectively clean the whole gingival embrasure (Fig. 5.5). Due to the design of the implant, embrasure space could be large in some cases. Interproximal brush would be a good modality to clean larger embrasure space and under multi-unit connector bars [52].

Waterfloss

Oral irrigators are a beneficial adjunct for interproximal cleaning and to remove biofilm around dental implants. They can be particularly useful to access hard-to-reach areas due to the emergence profiles of implants. Patients are advised to use oral irrigators rather than those with metal tips, which can scratch the implant surface. A study comparing oral irrigation and floss revealed that the Waterpik Water Flosser was 81% in reducing bleeding compared to 33% using floss. Excessive water pressure should not be used, and the flow of irrigation should be

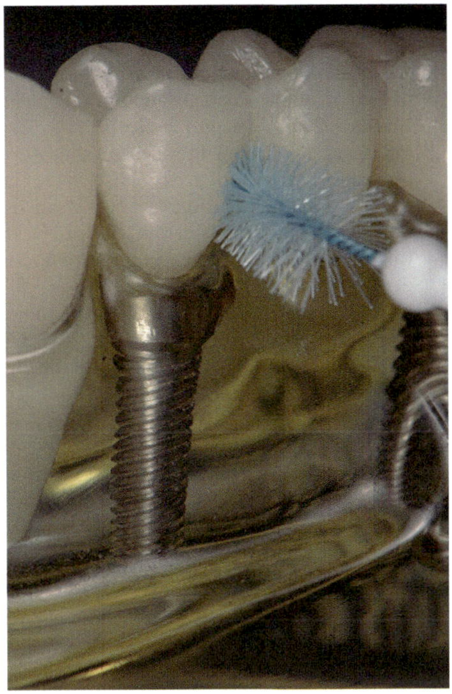

Fig. 5.5 A proper technique to use interproximal brush. Insert the brush interdentally while using a circular motion

aimed through the contact and not gingivally into the tissue. As an added benefit, chlorhexidine gluconate can be substituted for water for an antimicrobial effect [53–31].

Rubber Tip

A rubber tip stimulator can be an effective tool in interproximal cleaning and stimulating healthy gingiva. The patient is instructed to place the tip of the stimulator flat against the gingiva. With light pressure, the rubber tip is rolled interproximally. Light blanching is a sign of correct pressure. This device compresses interdental tissue against the implant prosthesis to help dislodge interproximal plaque [52].

5.6 Conclusion

As the number of patients receiving dental implant treatment is increasing, it is essential for providers and patients to know proper implant care and the challenges to maintaining peri-implant health. Constant maintenance by both parties and close monitoring of the peri-implant health are keys to ensure long-term success of the implant treatment.

References

1. Salvi GE, Zitzmann NU. The effects of anti-infective preventive measures on the occurrence of biologic implant complications and implant loss: a systematic review. Int J Oral Maxillofac Implants. 2014;29(Suppl):292–307.
2. Papathanasiou E, et al. Prevalence, etiology and treatment of peri-implant mucositis and peri-implantitis: a survey of periodontists in the United States. J Periodontol. 2016;87(5):493–501.
3. Derks J, Tomasi C. Peri-implant health and disease. A systematic review of current epidemiology. J Clin Periodontol. 2015;42(Suppl 16):S158–71.
4. Cosgarea R, et al. Prevalence of peri-implant diseases–a critical review on the current evidence. Braz Oral Res. 2019;33:e063.
5. Costa FO, et al. Peri-implant disease in subjects with and without preventive maintenance: a 5-year follow-up. J Clin Periodontol. 2012;39(2):173–81.
6. Berglundh T, Lindhe J, Ericsson I, Marinello CP, Liljenberg B, Thomsen P. The soft tissue barrier at implants and teeth. Clin Oral Implants Res. 1991;2:81–90.
7. Casado PL, et al. Is bleeding on probing a differential diagnosis between periimplant health and disease? Braz J Oral Sci. 2013;12(2):95–9.
8. Hashim D, et al. The diagnosis of peri-implantitis: a systematic review on the predictive value of bleeding on probing. Clin Oral Implants Res. 2018;29:276–93.
9. Cornelini R, et al. Vascular endothelial growth factor and microvessel density around healthy and failing dental implants. Int J Oral Maxillofac Implants. 2001;16(3):389.
10. Jepsen S, et al. Primary prevention of peri-implantitis: managing peri-implant mucositis. J Clin Periodontol. 2015;42:S152–7.
11. Smeets R, et al. Impact of dental implant surface modifications on osseointegration. Biomed Res Int. 2016;2016:6285620.
12. Dahiya V, Shukla P, Gupta S. Surface topography of dental implants: a review. J Dent Implants. 2014;4(1):66.
13. De Bruyn H, et al. Implant surface roughness and patient factors on long-term peri-implant bone loss. Periodontology 2000. 2017;73(1):218–27.
14. Todescan S, Lavigne S, Kelekis-Cholakis A. Guidance for the maintenance care of dental implants: clinical review. J Can Dent Assoc. 2012;78(1):107.
15. Teughels W, Van Assche N, Sliepen I, Quirynen M. Effect of material characteristics and/or surface topography on biofilm development. Clin Oral Implants Res. 2006;17(Suppl 2):68–81.
16. Salvi GE, Aglietta M, Eick S, Sculean A, Lang NP, Ramseier CA. Reversibil- ity of experimental peri-implant mucositis com- pared with experimental gingivitis in humans. Clin Oral Implants Res. 2012;23:182–90.
17. Salvi G, Ramseier C. Efficacy of patient- administered mechanical and/or chemical pla- que control protocols in the management of peri-implant mucositis. A systematic review. J Clin Periodontol. 2015;42(Suppl. 16):S187–201.
18. Schwarz F, Becker K, Sager M. Effi- cacy of professionally-administered plaque removal with or without adjunctive measures for the treatment of peri-implant mucositis. A systematic review and meta-analysis. J Clin Periodontol. 2015;42(Suppl. 16):S201–12.
19. Ramanauskaite A, Tervonen T. The efficacy of supportive peri-implant therapies in preventing peri-implantitis and implant loss: a systematic review of the literature. J Oral Maxillofac Res. 2016;7:3.
20. Serino G, Turri A, Lang NP. Maintenance therapy in patients following the surgical treatment of peri-implantitis: a 5-year follow-up study. Clin Oral Implants Res. 2015;26(8):950–6.
21. Schwarz F, et al. Peri-implantitis. J Clin Periodontol. 2018;45:S246–66.
22. Renvert S, et al. Diagnosis and non-surgical treatment of peri-implant diseases and maintenance care of patients with dental implants–consensus report of working group 3. Int Dent J. 2019;69:12–7.
23. Albrektsson T, et al. The long-term efficacy of currently used dental implants: a review and proposed criteria of success. Int J Oral Maxillofac Implants. 1986;1(1):11–25.

24. Gulati M, et al. Implant maintenance: a clinical update. Int Sch Res Notices. 2014;2014:908534.
25. Misch CE, editor. Contemporary implant dentistry. 3rd ed. Mosby, Elsevier; 2007. p. 1055–72; (chapter 41).
26. Lindhe J, Meyle J. Group D of European workshop on periodontology. Collaborators (13) peri-implant diseases: consensus report of the sixth European workshop on periodontology. J Clin Periodontol. 2008;35:282–5.
27. Gerber JA, et al. Bleeding on probing and pocket probing depth in relation to probing pressure and mucosal health around oral implants. Clin Oral Implants Res. 2009;20(1):75–8.
28. Lang NP, et al. Absence of bleeding on probing an indicator of periodontal stability. J Clin Periodontol. 1990;17(10):714–21.
29. Fox SC, Moriarty JD, Kusy RP. The effects of scaling a titanium implant surface with metal and plastic instruments: an in vitro study. J Periodontol. 1990;61(8):485–90.
30. Goldstein RE, Nimmons KJ. The expanding esthetic practice: implant maintenance—part 2. Contemp Esthet Restor Pract. 2005;1:2–25.
31. Cavitron Soft Tip Ultrasonic Implant Insert 30 kHz Each, Dentsply Sirona, https://www.henryschein.com/us-en/dental/p/small-equipment/power-scaling-tips-inserts/cavitron-softip-ultrasonic/1670005.
32. Graumann SJ, Sensat ML, Stoltenberg JL. Air polishing: a review of current literature. Am Dent Hyg Assoc. 2013;87(4):173–80.
33. Petersilka G, et al. Effect of glycine powder air-polishing on the gingiva. J Clin Periodontol. 2008;35(4):324–32.
34. Cohen RE. Research, science and therapy committee, American Academy of periodontology. Position paper: periodontal maintenance. J Periodontol. 2003;74(9):1395–401.
35. Home-American Dental Association. [cited 2019Dec21]. https://www.ada.org/en.
36. Subramani K, Jung RE, Molenberg A, Hämmerle CH. Biofilm on dental implants: a review of the literature. Int J Oral Maxillofac Implants. 2009;24(4):616.
37. Wingrove SS. Peri-implant therapy for the dental hygienist: clinical guide to maintenance and disease complications. John Wiley & Sons; 2013.
38. Bass CC. The optimum characteristics of toothbrushes for personal oral hygiene. Dent Items Interest. 1948;70(7):697–718.
39. Bass CC. An effective method of personal oral hygiene. J La State Med Soc. 1954;106(2):57.
40. Lang NP, Lindhe J, editors. Clinical periodontology and implant dentistry, 2 Volume Set. John Wiley & Sons; 2015.
41. Kracher CM. Oral health maintenance of dental implants. Dent Assist. 2010;79(2):27.
42. Esposito M, Worthington HV, Thomsen P, Coulthard P. Interventions for replacing missing teeth: maintaining health around dental implants. Cochrane Database Syst Rev. 2004;3:CD003069.
43. Moritis K, Jenkins W, Hefti A, Schmitt P, McGrady M. A randomized, parallel design study to evaluate the effects of a Sonicare and a manual toothbrush on plaque and gingivitis. J Clin Dent. 2008;19(2):64–8.
44. Pelka AK, Nagler T, Hopp I, Petschelt A, Pelka MA. Professional brushing study comparing the effectiveness of sonic brush heads with manual toothbrushes: a single blinded, randomized clinical trial. Clin Oral Investig. 2011;15(4):451–60.
45. Robinson P, Deacon SA, Deery C, Heanue M, Walmsley AD, Worthington HV, Glenny AM, Shaw BC. Manual versus powered toothbrushing for oral health. Cochrane Database Syst Rev. 2005;2:CD002281.
46. Sicilia A, Arregui I, Gallego M, Cabezas B, Cuesta S. A systematic review of powered vs. manual toothbrushes in periodontal cause-related therapy. J Clin Periodontol. 2002;29:39–54.
47. Tritten CB, Armitage GC. Comparison of a sonic and a manual toothbrush for efficacy in supra-gingival plaque removal and reduction of gingivitis. J Clin Periodontol. 1996;23(7):641–8.
48. der Weijden Van FA, Timmerman MF, Snoek IM, Reijerse E, der Velden VU. Toothbrushing duration and plaque removing efficacy of electric toothbrushes. Am J Dent. 1996;9:S31–6.
49. Warren PR, Ray TS, Cugini M, Chater BV. A practice-based study of a power toothbrush: assessment of effectiveness and acceptance. J Am Dent Assoc. 2000;131(3):389–94.

50. Hellstadius K, Åsman B, Gustafsson A. Improved maintenance of plaque control by electrical toothbrushing in periodontitis patients with low compliance. J Clin Periodontol. 1993;20(4):235–7.
51. Yukna RA. Optimizing clinical success with implants: maintenance and care. Compend Suppl. 1993;15:S554–61.
52. Lyle DM, Qaqish JG, Schuller R. Evaluation of the plaque removal efficacy of a water flosser compared to string floss in adults after a single use. J Clin Dent. 2013;24:37–42.
53. Gorur A, Lyle DM, Schaudinn C, Costerton JW. Biofilm removal with a dental water jet. Compend Contin Educ Dent. 2009;30:1–6.
54. Felo A, Shibly O, Ciancio SG, Lauciello FR, Ho A. Effects of subgingival chlorhexidine irrigation on peri-implant maintenance. Am J Dent. 1997;10(2):107–10.
55. Magnuson B, Harsono M, Silberstein J. Water flosser vs. floss: comparing reduction in bleeding around implants. J Dent Res. 2013;92:3761.

6 Management of Common Soft Tissue Pathology Around Dental Implants

Mansour Hamad Alaskar

6.1 Introduction

In 1965, an orthopedic surgeon, Branemark, installed the first titanium tooth implant on a human volunteer [1]. Then, the first immediate implant placement was accredited to Professor Wilfried Schulte in 1978 [2]. Since 1990, the placement of dental implants in the post-extraction site has been a subject of considerable concern in the field of implant density. The option of implant placement as a replacement for tooth loss became very common in the 1990s, motivated by the development of guided bone regeneration. The dental specialist has, however, started to concentrate steadily on the esthetic outcome of the post-extraction implant placement over the past years, and some reports have highlighted a substantial risk of experiencing mucosal recessions, soft and hard tissue pathology with dental implants. The aim of this chapter is to discuss the common soft tissue pathology around dental implants and its management. It is worth starting this chapter with the anatomical difference between peri-implant soft tissue and soft tissue around the tooth and common soft tissue pathology around dental implant etiology and elements considered for diagnosis and management to get the decision tree in determination of management protocol.

6.2 Peri-Implant Soft Tissue

The scientists explored the anatomical difference between peri-implant soft tissue and tooth soft tissue to better clarify the anatomical variations between the interface of tooth-soft tissue and implant-soft tissue. The soft tissue profile and care

M. H. Alaskar (✉)
Department of Periodontics and Community Dentistry, Institution, College of Dentistry, King Saud University, Riyadh, Saudi Arabia
e-mail: Malaskar@ksu.edu.sa

M. Hassan (ed.), *Peri-Implant Soft Tissue Management*,
https://doi.org/10.1007/978-3-031-45516-2_6

around implants is significantly more complicated than around teeth for three primary factors:

1. Marginal mucosal area.
2. Attachment of connective tissues.
3. The vascular supply gaps.

The measurements of the supracrustal gingival tissue (SGT) [3] (initially called biological width) are close to those present on the natural tooth and vary from 3 to 4 mm. The junctional epithelium is around 2 mm in length, and the connective tissue is nearly 1–1.5 mm. It binds to the implant and contains collagen fiber bundles, some of which invest in the periosteum of the bone crest and run a course parallel with the surface of the implant with more collagen and fewer fibroblasts. The three main sources of blood supply around the natural tooth are the following:

(a) The supraperiosteal vessels which supply the free and attached gingiva.
(b) Blood vessels from the periodontal ligament.
(c) Blood vessels from the alveolar bone.

The essential blood vessels from the periodontal ligament are absent in the case of implants. The single source of blood was from the supraperiosteal vessel at the alveolar bone periosteum. There is also a hypovascular–hypocellular connective tissue zone around the implant that is not found around natural tooth and more vulnerable to the inflammatory response [3] (Fig. 6.1).

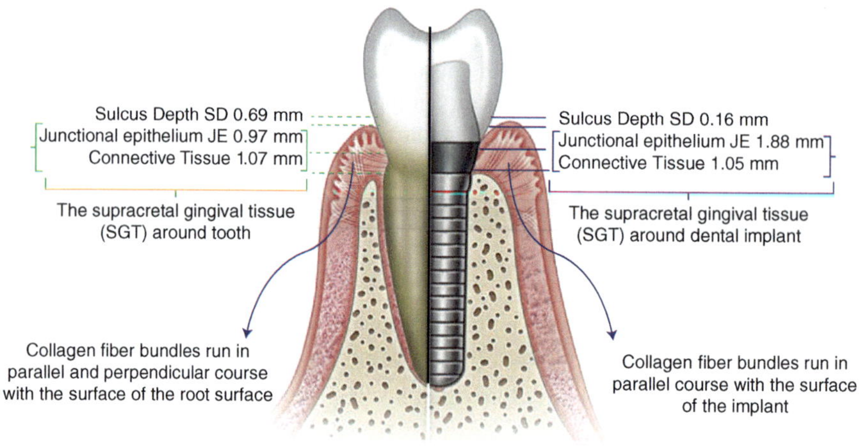

Fig. 6.1 Schematic drawing presenting the difference of the supracrustal gingival tissue (SGT) around tooth and implant

6.3 Peri-Implant Soft Tissue Importance

The mucosa surrounding the dental implant forms tight gingival cuff consisting of epithelium and connective tissues established during healing after the surgery [4]. Multiple findings have evidence on comparisons and variations at the dent–gingival junction between peri-implant soft tissue and gingiva around natural tooth [5–7] (Table 6.1).

Table 6.1 Distinctions between soft tissue peri-implant and gingiva around the teeth

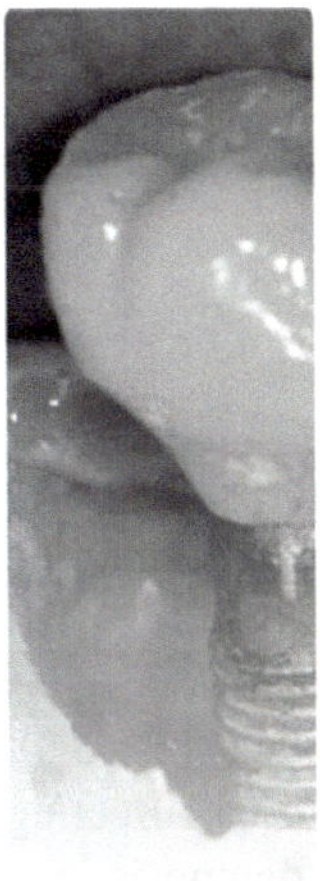

	Tooth	Implant
connection	Cementum, bone, PDL	OI(functional ankylosis), noPDL
JE	Hemidesmosomes& Basal lamina	Hemidesmosomes& Basal lamina
CT	Perpendicular fiber	Parallel fiber, CT cuff, no attachment
Vascularity	More	**less may have impaired defense capacity**
PD	3 in heath	2.5-4 (depended on ST depth)
BOP	More reliable	**less reliable**
	Cargiulo(1961)	**Cochran (1997)**
Sulcus Depth (SD)	0.69 mm	0.16 mm
JE	0.97 mm	1.88 mm
CT	1.07 mm	1.05 mm
BW	2.04 (JE+CT)	3.08 (JE+CT+BW)
	Probe Position	
Erricsson&Lindhe 1993	Health 1-2 mm to bone crest, coronal to apical part of JE	Health 0.2 mm to bone crest, Deep in CT, apical to CEJ
Schou (2002)	In health, broping similar b/w teeth & implants with inflammation, probing much deeper at implants	

JE junctional epithelium, *CT* connective tissue, *PD* probing depth, *BOP* bleeding on probing

6.4 Etiology of the Common Soft Tissue Pathology Around Dental Implants

Three main categories cause the soft tissue pathology around dental implants, broadly classified as inflammatory, reactive, and autoimmune [8]. The inflammatory group is characterized by two major conditions of the inflamed peri-implant tissues and its underlying supporting bone: peri-implant mucositis and peri-implantitis [9]. Reactive lesions in the oral cavity primarily include pyogenic granuloma (PG), peripheral giant cell granuloma (PGCG), and fibrous hyperplasia [10]. Lastly, oral lichens planus, an autoimmune mucocutaneous inflammatory disease, should be considered [11].

6.5 Inflammatory Conditions That Cause Soft Tissue Pathology Around Dental Implants and Bone Loss

6.5.1 Peri-Implant Mucositis and Peri-Implantitis

Peri-implant mucositis is defined as a reversible inflammation in the soft tissues surrounding the implant, which constitute the main common soft tissue pathology around the dental implant (Fig. 6.2). The advanced/progressive form of it is peri-implantitis, which involves the soft and hard tissue component and defined as inflammation associated with loss of supporting bone around an implant (Fig. 6.3). This section of the chapter will focus on these common two conditions affecting soft and hard tissue around the dental implant in terms of etiology, diagnosis, and management.

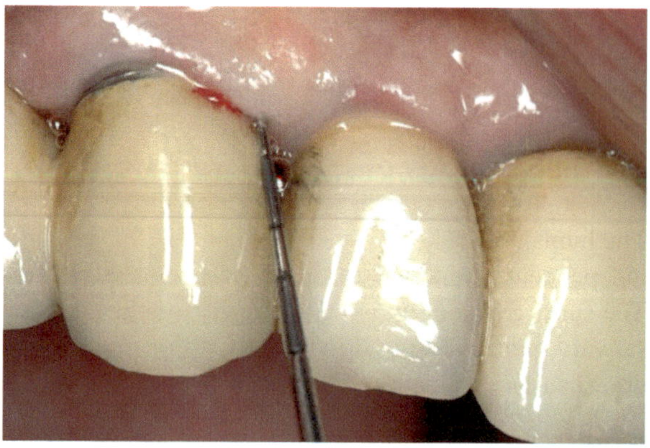

Fig. 6.2 Clinical photograph showing the peri-implant mucositis of the implant-supported crown in the upper right canine area characterized by normal probing depth with bleeding on probing (BOP)

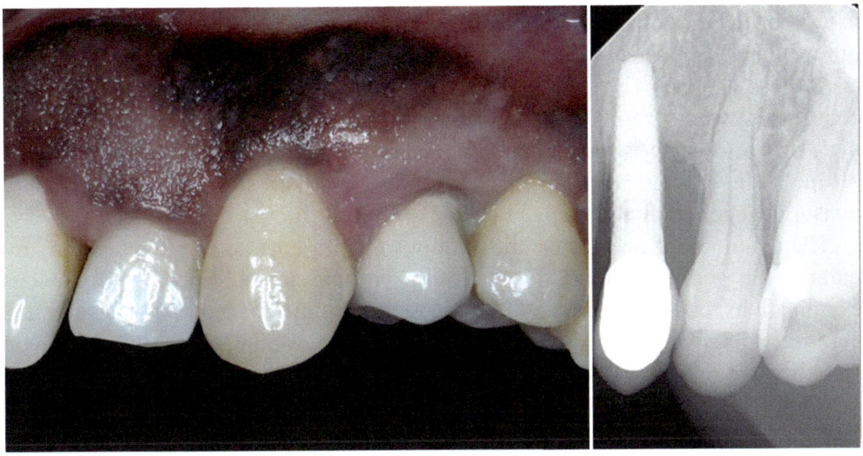

Fig. 6.3 Clinical photograph showing the peri-implantitis of the implant-supported crown in the upper left first premolar area characterized by progressive bone loss

6.5.2 Etiological and Risk Factors

The main etiology of both conditions is bacterial biofilm on the implant and restorations. However, many other multifactorial risk factors have been documented in the literature and attributed to the following: smoking, residual cement, trauma from occlusion, width and thickness of keratinized mucosa, foreign body reaction, untreated periodontal diseases, type of implant surface, genetic trait, lack of compliance, psychological reasons, and systematic diseases [12].

There is also evidence for radiation therapy as a risk indicator for peri-implant mucositis [13]. There is some evidence for diabetes mellitus as a risk indicator for peri-implant mucositis [14, 15]. Poorly controlled diabetes mellitus (HbA1c levels > 10.1) was shown to be associated with increased bleeding on probing at implants [15]. Ferreira et al. [16] also reported an association with peri-implant mucositis and systemic disease. However, the systemic diseases described included "diabetes mellitus, hormonal changes, menopause, chemotherapy, thyroid alterations, cardiac problems, and alcohol use," and thus the results of the study are difficult to interpret.

6.5.3 Diagnosis Criteria

The main clinical characteristics of peri-implant mucositis include bleeding on gentle probing; erythema, swelling, and/or suppuration may also be present. An increase in probing depth is often observed in the presence of peri-implant mucositis because of swelling or a decrease in probing resistance, which needs to be considered to avoid misdiagnosis. The absence of bone loss beyond crestal-bone-level changes, confirmed by radiographs, indicates alterations resulting from initial bone remodeling. There is strong evidence from animal and human experimental studies that plaque is the etiological factor for peri-implant mucositis and can be resolved by nonsurgical periodontal therapy [17].

The diagnosis of peri-implantitis requires the presence of bleeding and/or suppuration on gentle probing, an increase in probing depth compared to previous examinations, and the presence of bone loss beyond the crestal bone levels. In the absence of previous examination data, diagnosis of peri-implantitis can be based on the combination of the following: the presence of bleeding and/or suppuration on gentle probing, probing depths of ≥6 mm, and bone levels ≥3 mm apical to the most coronal portion of the intra-osseous part of the implant [18].

6.5.4 Treatment of Peri-Implant Mucositis and Peri-Implantitis

Peri-implant mucositis is primarily caused by a disruption of the host–microbe homeostasis at the implant–mucosa interface and is a reversible condition at the host biomarker level. Regular supportive peri-implant therapy with biofilm removal is an important first preventive strategy against the conversion of health to peri-implant mucositis and also against the progression of peri-implant mucositis to peri-implantitis [17].

In addition to the biofilm removal, it is very substantial to determine the goal of therapy for both peri-implant mucositis and peri-implantitis, which is usually confined to control of the bacterial etiology, elimination of soft tissue inflammation, implant surface decontamination, regenerative approach, resective approach, implant surface modification (implantoplasty), and re-osseointegration [19].

Furthermore, it is important to take into consideration the limitations of the therapy, ranging from accessibility, implant configuration, implant surface structure, soft tissue conditions, defect configuration, and grafting materials to the amount of bone loss [20, 21].

As mentioned earlier, biofilm removal by nonsurgical mechanical debridement (MD) is the first treatment procedure for the treatment of peri-implant mucositis along with local chemotherapeutic antiseptic agents. There are numerous therapies, such as antibiotic and probiotic therapy, laminin coatings on implant surfaces, low-level laser therapy, and photodynamic therapy (PDT), that have been assessed as adjuncts to MD for the treatment of peri-implant diseases [22–27].

Photodynamic therapy (PDT) is another form of local therapy that has been used as an adjunct to MD for peri-implant diseases in several studies [23, 28–31]. In this form of adjunct therapy, a dye (photosensitizer) is locally delivered to the peri-implant sulci of infected sites and is then exposed to a laser with a wavelength usually ranging between 660 to 800 nm [32]. The resultant reaction produces reactive oxygen species (ROS), which possibly reduce inflammation and counts of pathogenic microbes at the treatment sites, thereby facilitating the overall healing process. Studies [29, 33] have explored the contribution of PDT as an aide treatment to routine oral hygiene maintenance instructions for the treatment of periodontal and peri-implant diseases. It has also been proposed that MD with adjunct PDT is more effective in reducing peri-implant soft tissue inflammation (peri-implant mucositis) than MD alone [34].

In cases of peri-implant mucositis, the etiology attributed to the lack of keratinized tissue (KT) surgical periodontal treatment, including gingival graft after the phase of MD, is considered. Although there was debate in the dental literature about the prevalence of peri-implant soft tissue diseases and lack of KT, an increase in the width of KT may be considered in order to improve and simplify the patient's oral hygiene and to preserve the level of mucosal tissue [35–37]. For dental implants and natural teeth alike, the value of having an acceptable width and density of KT tends to be important, comparably to teeth without KT, which were observed to be more vulnerable to more impairment of attachment [38]. Tissue breakdown has also been found to develop more rapidly with dental implants than with teeth [39] (Figs. 6.4 and 6.5).

Peri-implant mucositis, the most common soft tissue pathology around dental implants, seems to be a precursor to subsequent peri-implantitis. The treatment during the transitional stage typically involves antibacterial therapy, combined with

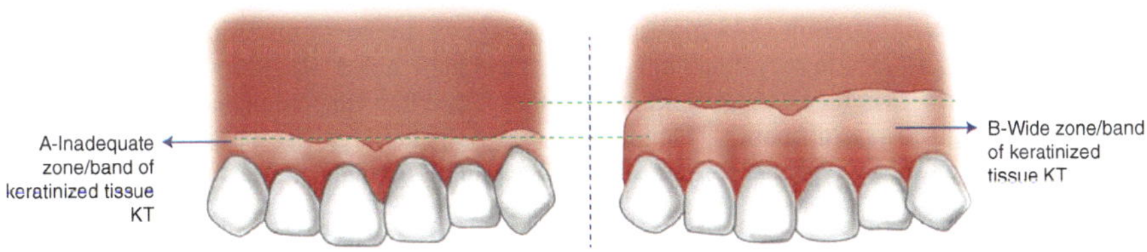

Fig. 6.4 Schematic drawing presenting the differences between A inadequate zone of keratinized tissue (KT) and B wide zone of KT

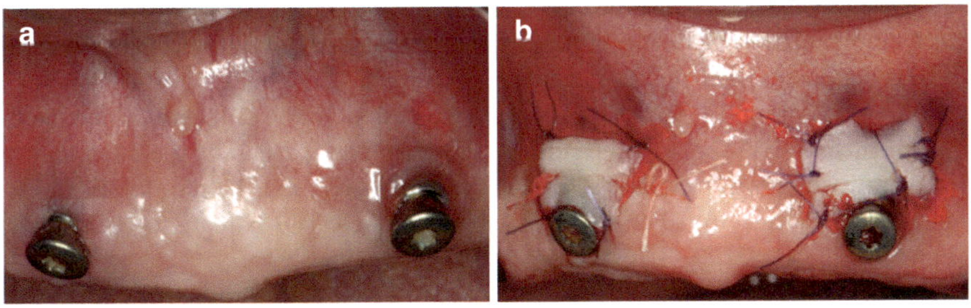

Fig. 6.5 (**a**) Labial view of a two-implant-supported overdenture with a lack of keratinized attached gingiva and peri-implant mucositis. (**b**) Free gingival graft done around a two-implant-supported overdenture to increase the zone of keratinized attached gingiva and enhance patient oral hygiene practice

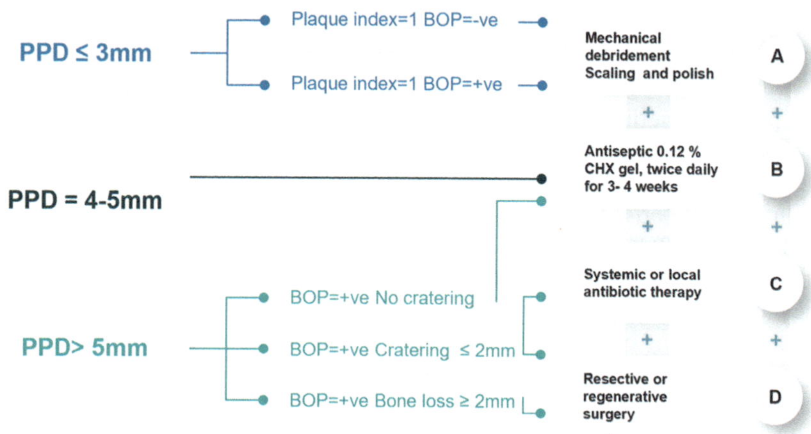

Fig. 6.6 Cumulative Interceptive Supportive Therapy (CIST) by Lang 1997. Depending on peri-implant probing depth (PDD), plaque index, bleeding on probing (BOP), and cratering with guided four treatment options according to the clinical and radiographic findings. Treatment A is mechanical cleansing using rubber cups, polishing paste, and acrylic sealers for chipping-off calculus. Instruction for more effective oral hygiene practices, Treatment B is antiseptic therapy. Rinses with 0.1–0.2% chlorhexidine digluconate for 30 s using approximately 10 mL, for 3–4 weeks supplemented by irrigating locally with chlorhexidine (preferably 0.2–0.5%) using a Luer syringe or local chlorhexidine gel application. Treatment C is antibiotic therapy 1-systemic ornidazol (2 × 500 mg/die) or metronidazole (2 × 250 mg/die) for 10 days or a combination of metronidazole (500 mg/die) plus amoxicillin (375 mg/die) for 10 days. 2. Local: Application of slow-release devices for 10 days (25% tetracycline fibers). D Surgical approach 1. Regenerative surgery using abundant saline rinses at the defect, barrier membranes, close flap adaptation, and careful postsurgical monitoring for several months. Plaque control is to be assured by applying chlorhexidine gels. 2. Resective surgery. Apically repositioning of the flap following osteoplasty around the defect

MD before attempting surgical regeneration of peri-implant alveolar bone lost due to infection. Lang et al. in 1997 [40] published a review of clinical trials on therapies for peri-implant infections, revealing that the inflammatory process in soft and mineralized peri-implant tissues can be controlled. This renders the site susceptible to regenerative procedures aimed at re-establishing osseointegration after nonsurgical therapy and the administration of local and systematic antibiotics. However, as of today, no controlled studies have been performed to document the possibility of true osseointegration [20, 41, 42]. A previous cited study [40] proposed a well-documented system for the management of peri-implant diseases called cumulative interceptive supportive therapy (CIST). This approach is very helpful for the development of a joint effort for the management of soft and hard tissue conditions (Fig. 6.6).

Surgical treatment therapy for peri-implantitis, as it is the progressive disease of the common soft tissue pathology around dental implants, is mainly a regenerative approach [43]. The treatment consisted of flap reflection, surface decontamination, use of enamel matrix derivative (EMD) or platelet-derived growth factor (PDGF), and guided bone regeneration with mineralized freeze-dried bone and/or anorganic bovine bone combined with PDGF or EMD and covered with an absorbable membrane and/or subepithelial connective tissue graft (Fig. 6.7).

However, the destructive soft tissue pathological inflammatory process affects both soft and hard tissues, leading to pocket formation and progressive bone

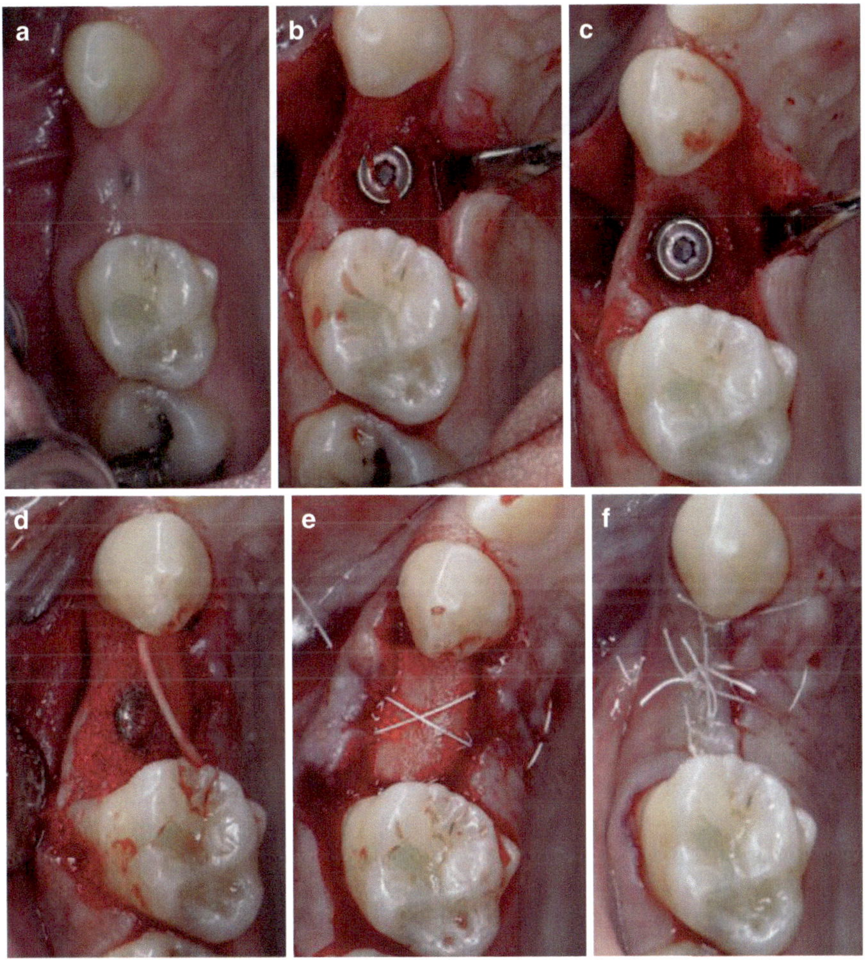

Fig. 6.7 Soft tissue fistula around the implant of upper right first premolar with bone loss. (**a**) Pre-surgical view showing the soft tissue fistula. (**b**) surgical view showing the soft tissue granulation around the dental implant. (**c**) Surgical view showing the bone loss and defect around the dental implant after degranulation. (**d**) Peri-implant bone graft with a membrane around contained bony defects of the implant. (**e**) Membrane adaption above the bone graft and implant. (**f**) Primary coverage with EPTF suture. (**g**) Second stage and connection of the healing abutment after 4 months post-surgical. (**h**) Pre-surgical radiograph showed mesial and distal vertical bone loss around the dental implant. (**i**) Post-surgical radiograph after bone graft. (**j**) 4 months post-surgical bone graft showed bony filled

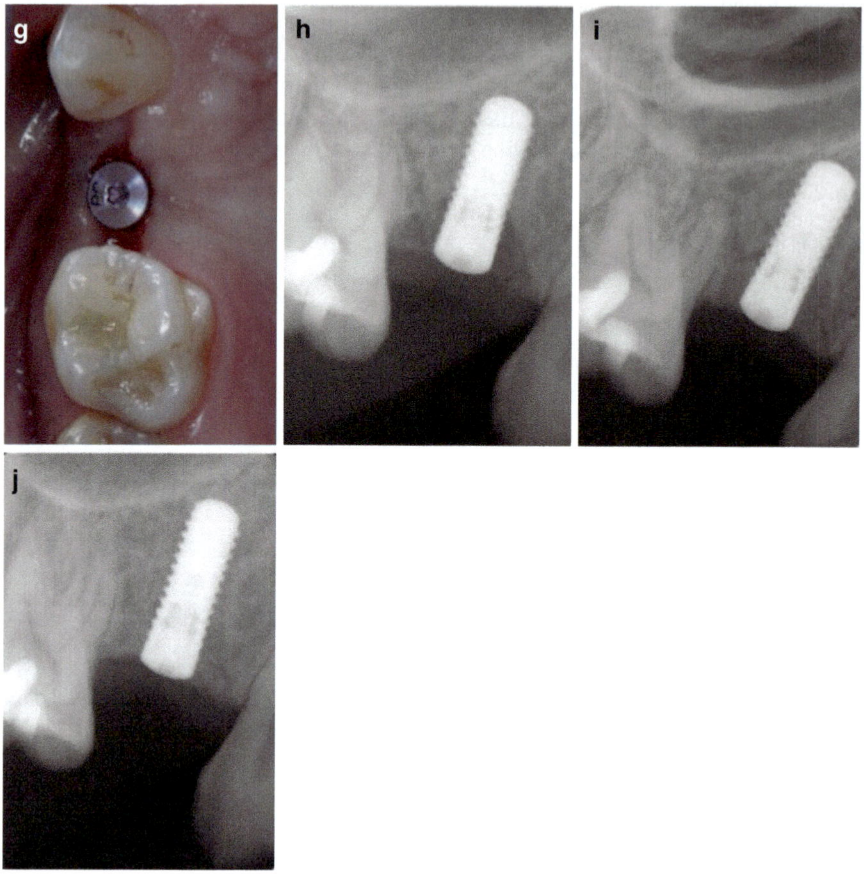

Fig. 6.7 (continued)

resorption around osseointegrated oral implants. Explanation may be indicated in advanced stages with severe bone loss when soft tissue pathology cannot be eradicated with re-augmentation of the site for new implant placement and restoration (Fig. 6.8) [44].

According to published studies [16, 45], peri-implant diseases are very common. Therefore, it is imperative for the clinician to examine and evaluate patients who have been provided with implant-supported restorations on a regular basis.

The following aspects are recommended for the clinical routine:

When implant treatment is considered, patients should be informed of the risks for biological complications (peri-implant diseases) and the need for preventive care. An individual risk assessment, including systemic and local risk indicators, should be performed, and modifiable risk factors, such as residual increased probing pocket depth in the remaining dentition or smoking, should be eliminated. Hence, treatment of periodontal disease aiming for elimination of residual pockets with bleeding on probing and smoking cessation should precede implant placement [46].

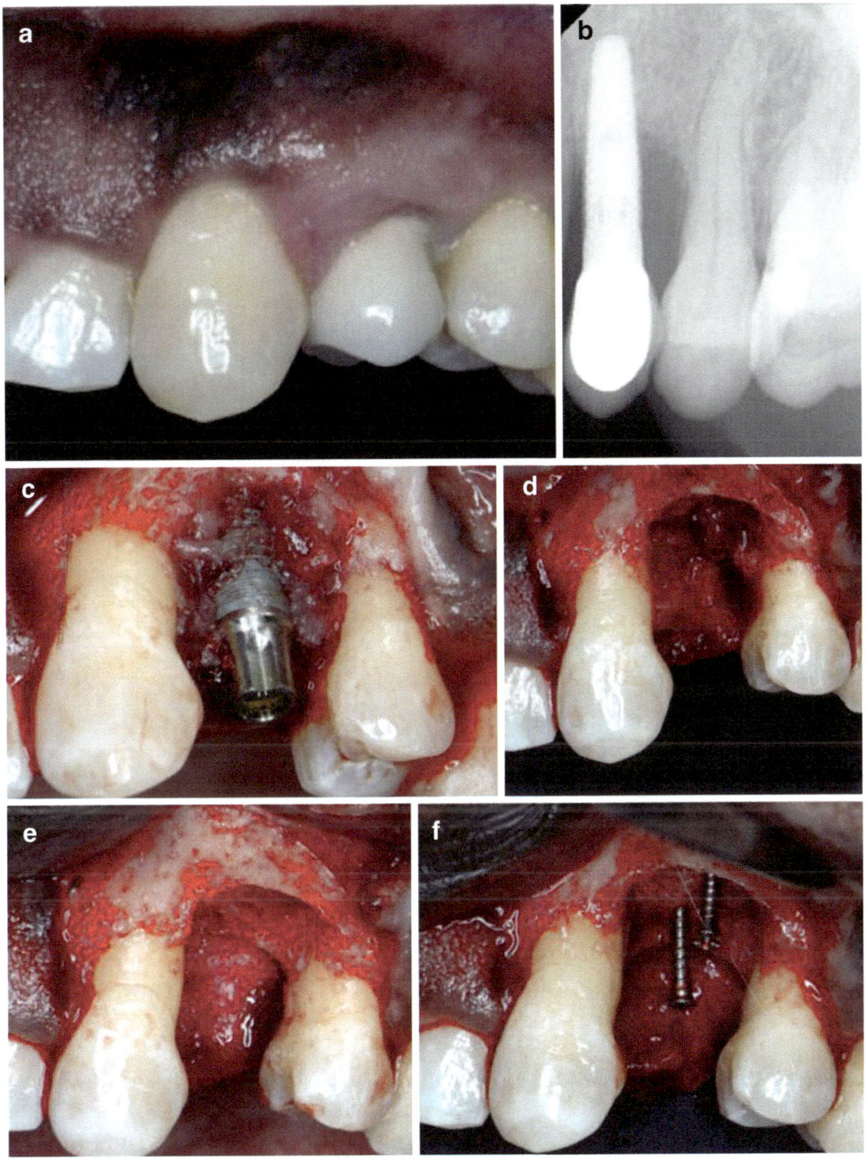

Fig. 6.8 Destructive soft tissue pathological inflammatory process affects both soft and hard tissues, leading to implant failure of the area of the upper left first premolar. (**a**) Pre-surgical view showing the soft tissue inflammation and rolled margin. (**b**) Pre-surgical radiograph showing an extensive amount of more than 50%. (**c**) Surgical view showing the pathological soft granulation tissue around the dental implant. (**d**) Surgical view after implant explanation. (**e**) Surgical view after complete soft tissue degranulation. (**f**) Surgical view with two tenting screws to vertically augment the alveolar bone. (**g**) Radiograph showing labial and palatal vertical tenting screw. (**h**) Surgical view after bone graft. (**i**) Surgical view after membrane adaption. (**j**) Occlusal view after suture and achieving primary coverage. (**k**) Labial view after suture and achieving primary coverage

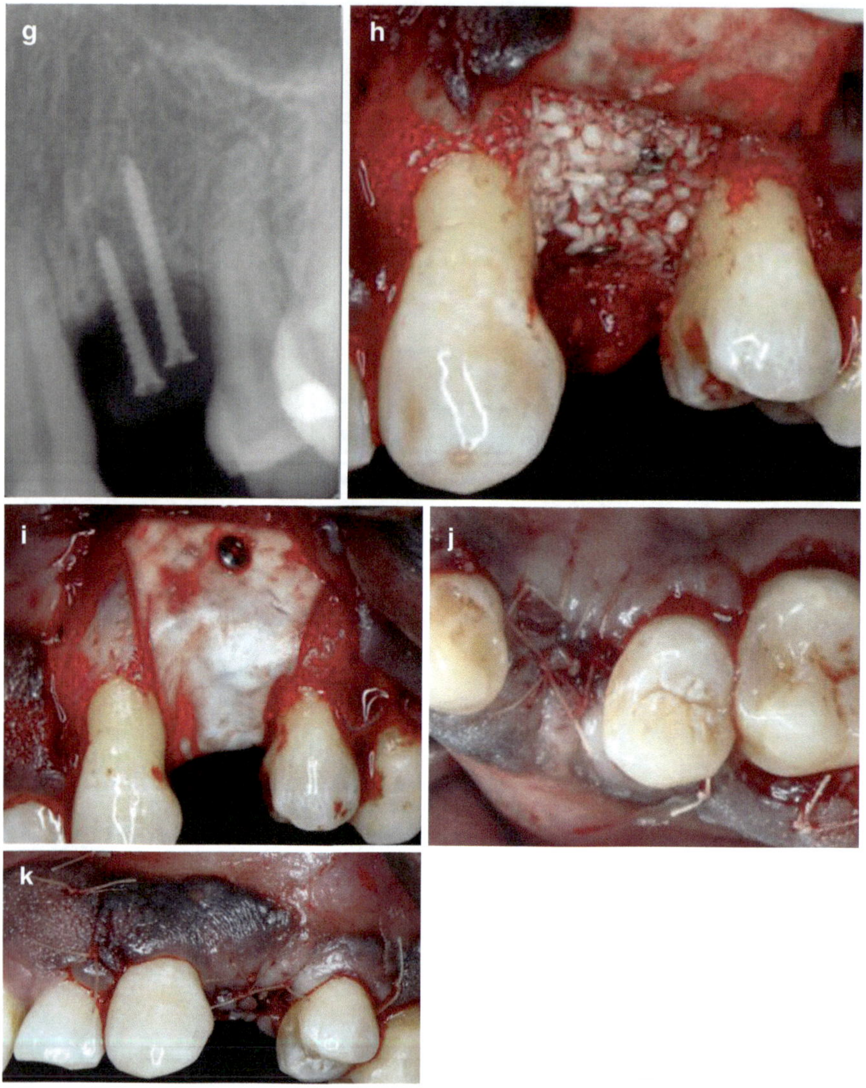

Fig. 6.8 (continued)

The correct fit of implant components and the superstructures has to be ensured to avoid additional niches for biofilm adherence [47]. If cemented implant restorations have been selected, the restoration margins should be located at the mucosal margin in order to allow meticulous removal of excess cement [48, 49].

To facilitate personal oral hygiene, clinicians should consider having keratinized attached surrounding the transmucosal implant portion already during implant placement (for one-stage implant placement) or during abutment connection (for two-stage implant placement) [50].

Professional supportive care should be established according to the individual needs of the patient (e.g., 3, 6, or 12-month recall intervals), and their compliance has to be confirmed [51, 52]. Particularly in patients with a history of aggressive periodontitis indicating an increased susceptibility for periodontal and peri-implant diseases, shorter recall intervals should be considered. During recall, peri-implant tissues must be regularly examined, including probing assessments with special emphasis on bleeding on probing [12].

6.6 Reactive Condition That Causes Soft Tissue Pathology Around Dental Implants and Bone Loss

6.6.1 Pyogenic Granuloma

Pyogenic granuloma is a common, reactive inflammatory hyperplasia of the oral cavity. Although the term "pyogenic" is used, PG is not an infectious lesion. PG usually occurs as a response to different stimulating factors such as local trauma or irritation and iatrogenic and hormonal factors [10, 53]. Because of the female hormone factor, it has a very high incidence in young females, principally in the second decade of life. Clinically, PG presents as a painless, smooth, or lobulated shape. It is classed as a hemorrhagic lesion because of its vascular structure, and its color ranges from pink to dark red. It is presented clinically as sessile with an average size of 1 cm and has a smooth, shiny surface. In addition, it bleeds very easily when touched. Sometimes, its surface may be covered by a pseudo-membrane due to secondary ulcerations [54].

It was reported that oral PG was found in 18% of patients who had benign oral masses. It was also noted that PG can be observed in individuals as young as 10 years old up to the age of 70 [55]. It is the second most common soft tissue pathology around dental implants after peri-implant mucositis, soft tissue fistula, and peri-implantitis. As mentioned previously, local trauma is the main etiological factor, with 30–50% of patients with PG having a history of local trauma. The occurrence of implant related PG was associated with inappropriate healing caps of implants [56] (Fig. 6.9).

Biopsy as a diagnostic approach is warranted because peripheral odontogenic lesions, benign and malignant neoplasms, metastatic lesions, and a variety of other lesions may clinically resemble this reactive nodular lesion of the gingiva. The histopathologic analysis of PG usually reveals an intense vascular proliferation with extensive areas of ulceration, mixed inflammatory infiltrate, numerous granulation tissue, and abundant macrophages (multinucleated giant cells) [57] (Fig. 6.9c).

There are several treatment options for PG, such as surgical excision, cryotherapy, electro-cauterization, laser applications, and steroid injections [56]. However,

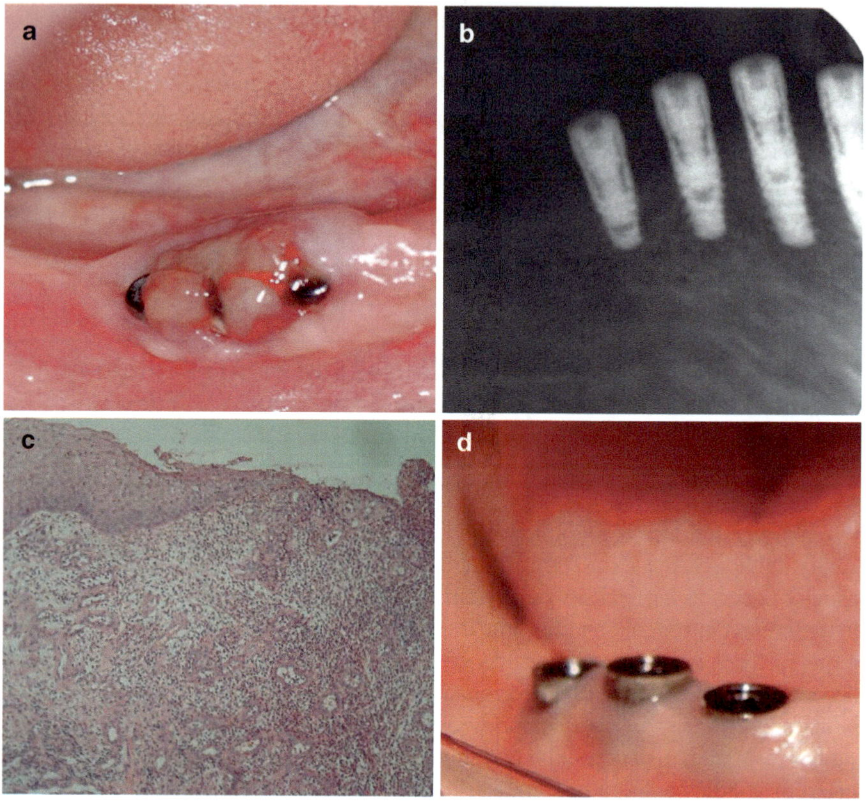

Fig. 6.9 Pyogenic granuloma around a dental implant [with permissions from Dr. Emrah Soylu]. (**a**) Clinical view of PG around a dental implant, 1 month after implant placement. (**b**) Peri-apical radiograph of the affected site. (**c**) In the upper left side of the section, the surface epithelium shows regenerative changes. Other sides of the epithelium are ulcerative. Leak connective tissue with edema, proliferative capillary vessels, and aggregation of active-chronic inflammatory cells can be seen at the bottom line of ulceration and in the subepithelial side (hematoxylin and eosin; original magnification 100×). (**d**) 3 months after the PG surgical removal

providing adequate keratinized soft tissue should be the first step to prevent such lesions for reactive lesions related to dental implants. In addition, management should involve the detection and elimination of the possible local irritant factors, such as abnormal superstructure and healing cap implant relationships or unfavorable implant–bone relationships. Soft tissue site preparation with gingival graft augmentation before implant placement is necessary to enhance the thickness and width of the keratinized gingiva when there is inadequate gingiva thickness and a lack of keratinization (Fig. 6.10) [57].

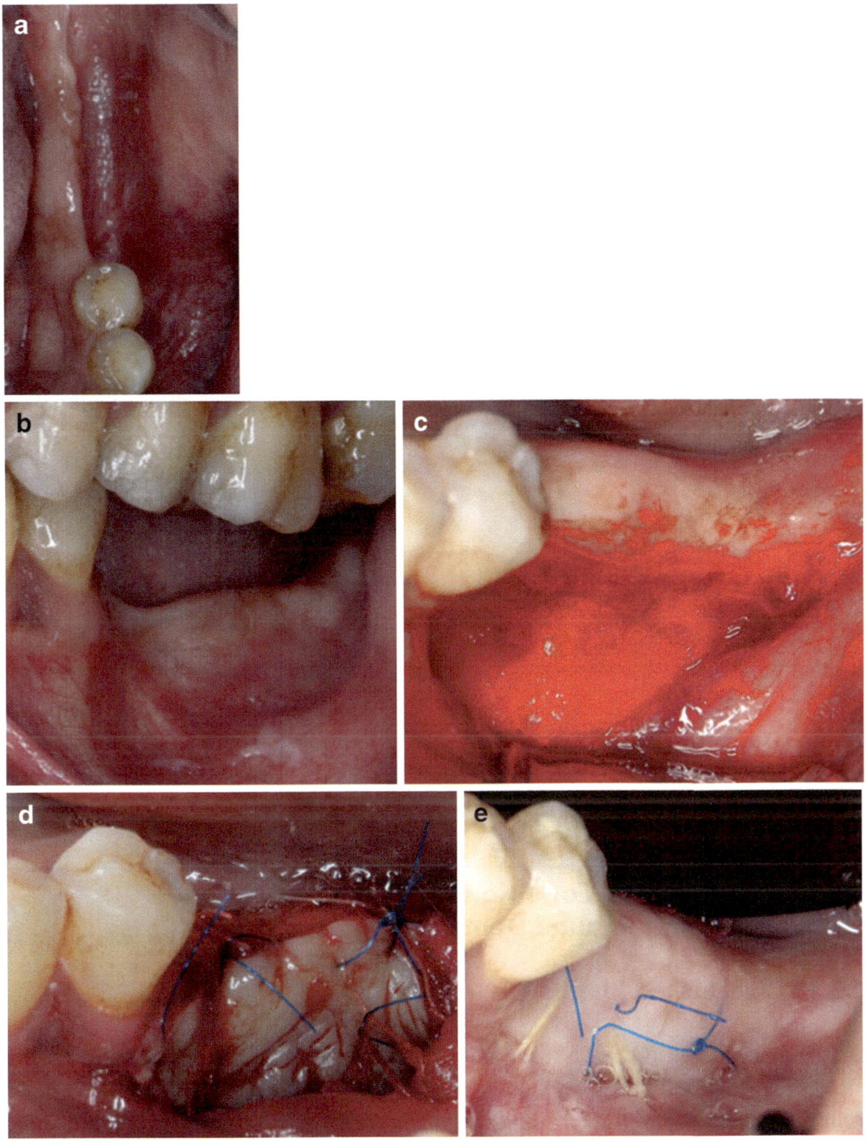

Fig. 6.10 Free gingiva graft with apical position flap and vestibuloplasty to increase zone of attached gingiva before ridge augmentation of lower left missing first and second molars. (**a**) Pre-surgical occlusal view showing a lack of keratinized attached gingiva. (**b**) Pre-surgical lateral view. (**c**) Surgical view showing the recipient site preparation. (**d**) Surgical view showing donor tissue FGG suturing and adapted in the recipient site. (**e**) 2 weeks post-surgically before suture removal. (**f**) Post-surgical occlusal view showing the amount of keratinized attached gingiva gain. (**g**) Post-surgical lateral view indicating the zone of attached gingiva in preparation for guided bone regeneration followed by future implant placement

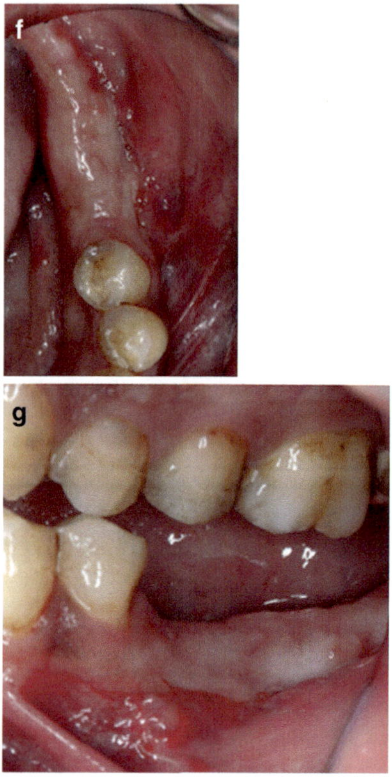

Fig. 6.10 (continued)

6.7 Autoimmune Conditions That Cause Soft Tissue Pathology Around Dental Implants and Bone Loss

6.7.1 Oral Lichen Planus

Oral lichen planus (OLP) is a chronic mucocutaneous inflammatory disease. It affects the skin, nails, hair, and mucous membranes (oral and genital) [58]. It most commonly affects middle-aged individuals, predominantly females [59]. Its prevalence is between 0.1% and 2.2% [60]. OLP is a T cell-mediated autoimmune disorder of uncertain etiology [58, 61]. Besides immune dysregulation, many etiological factors may also be involved, including traumatic insults, medication, dental materials, and stress [62]. It commonly affects buccal mucosa, tongue, and gingiva [63].

Due to the adverse effects of implant placement on LP and vice versa, implant placement should be done with caution [64]. LP patients treated with dental implants are at a risk of implant failure due to the inability of the epithelium to attach to the implant surface, which allows the bacteria to access the preimplant tissue, leading to the failure of osseointegration [65]. It has also been recommended that lichen planus patients be handled with care during the remission phase when the cases are stabilized [66]. It should not be placed during the active phase of the LP, which will cause implant failure (Fig. 6.11).

Corticosteroids are the main treatment for symptomatically OLP [67]. Topical steroids are considered first-line treatment because they are more effective in treating superficial inflammation, especially in EOLP [59]. Other treatment modalities are being tried to increase the efficacy and decrease the complications of corticosteroids. The therapeutic potential of photodynamic therapy [68] and lasers [69] has been investigated. Ozone therapy is also being used to treat OLP due to its strong antimicrobial activity [67]. Oral corticosteroid dose of 4 mg/daily after insertion of dental implants in patients with suppressed OLP to ensure suppression of the activated immune system is required as an element of the supportive implant therapy (SIT) [70] [Fig. 6.12].

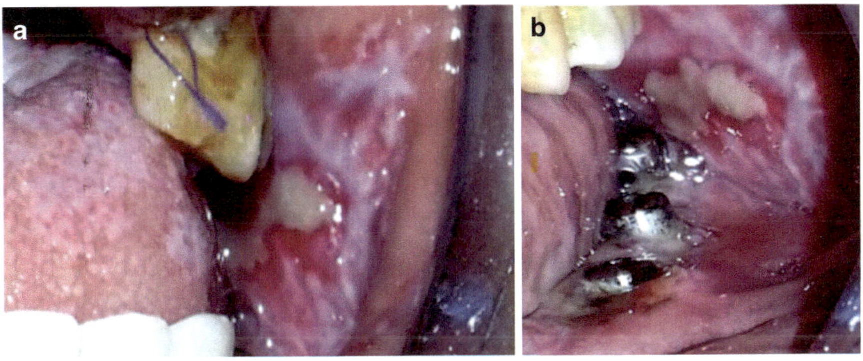

Fig. 6.11 Active phase of oral lichens planus with implant failure. (**a**) Clinical view of white striation and ulceration of a patient suffering from active lichen planus. (**b**) Failed implants placed into a patient suffering from active lichen planus. (With permission from Dr. Moustafa Abboushelib)

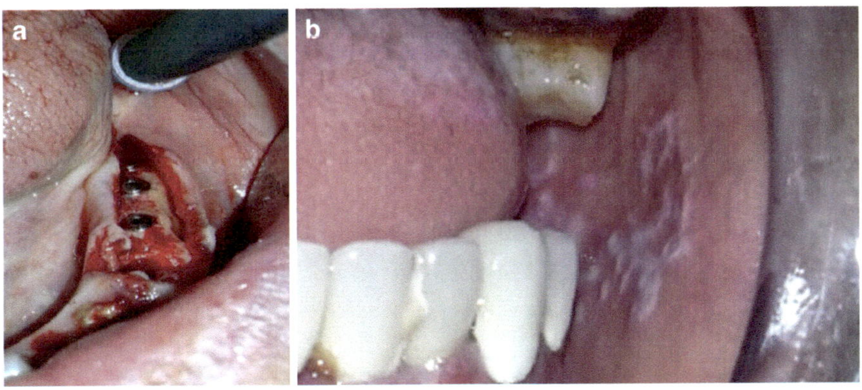

Fig. 6.12 Active phase of oral lichens planus with implant failure. (**a**) Surgical view of insertion of submerged implants after application of systemic corticosteroids and soft tissue laser irradiation. Notice the complete disappearance of soft tissue symptoms. (**b**) Implant-supported restoration after 3 years in function. Notice the recurrence of some white striation. (With permission from Dr. Moustafa Abboushelib)

6.8 Conclusion

An adequate treatment plan and supportive periodontal and implant therapy, along with proper oral hygiene care, are the keys to the success of dental implant treatment. However, just like its natural predecessor, a dental implant may be subject to destructive soft and hard tissue pathology. Soft tissue pathology is the first sign of peri-implant diseases. Therefore, in the case of peri-implant soft tissue pathology, the knowledge of the accurate etiology as inflammatory, reactive, or autoimmune is essential to formulating the treatment goals of each clinical case situation. Following the decision trees at the end of this chapter will facilitate the platform form in the field of dental implant practice (Fig. 6.13).

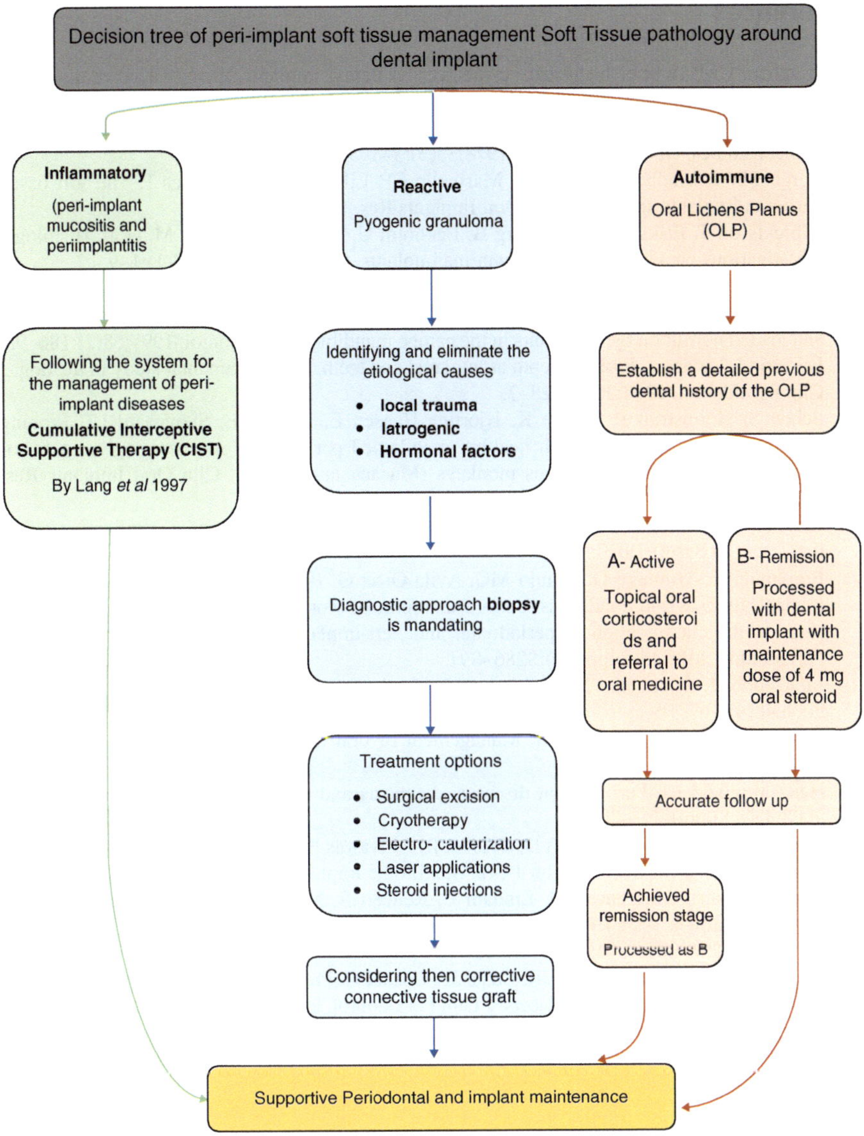

Fig. 6.13 Decision tree showing the treatment objective and option of the soft tissue pathology around the dental implant

References

1. Abraham CM. A brief historical perspective on dental implants, their surface coatings and treatments. Open Dent J. 2014;8:50–5.
2. Schulte W, Kleineikenscheidt H, Lindner K, Schareyka R. The Tubingen immediate implant in clinical studies. Dtsch Zahnarztl Z. 1978;33(5):348–59.
3. Berglundh T, Lindhe J, Ericsson I, Marinello CP, Liljenberg B, Thomsen P. The soft tissue barrier at implants and teeth. Clin Oral Implants Res. 1991;2(2):81–90.
4. Albrektsson T, Eriksson AR, Friberg B, Lekholm U, Lindahl L, Nevins M, et al. Histologic investigations on 33 retrieved nobelpharma implants. Clin Mater. 1993;12(1):1–9.
5. Cochran DL, Hermann JS, Schenk RK, Higginbottom FL, Buser D. Biologic width around titanium implants. A histometric analysis of the implanto-gingival junction around unloaded and loaded nonsubmerged implants in the canine mandible. J Periodontol. 1997;68(2):186–98.
6. Ericsson I, Lindhe J. Probing depth at implants and teeth. An experimental study in the dog. J Clin Periodontol. 1993;20(9):623–7.
7. Schou S, Holmstrup P, Stoltze K, Hjorting-Hansen E, Fiehn NE, Skovgaard LT. Probing around implants and teeth with healthy or inflamed peri-implant mucosa/gingiva. A histologic comparison in cynomolgus monkeys (Macaca fascicularis). Clin Oral Implants Res. 2002;13(2):113–26.
8. Khan A, Sharma D. Management of peri-implant diseases: a survey of Australian periodontists. Dent J (Basel). 2020;8(3):100.
9. Berglundh T, Armitage G, Araujo MG, Avila-Ortiz G, Blanco J, Camargo PM, et al. Peri-implant diseases and conditions: consensus report of workgroup 4 of the 2017 world workshop on the classification of periodontal and Peri-implant diseases and conditions. J Clin Periodontol. 2018;45(Suppl 20):S286–S91.
10. Jafarzadeh H, Sanatkhani M, Mohtasham N. Oral pyogenic granuloma: a review. J Oral Sci. 2006;48(4):167–75.
11. Scully C, Eisen D, Carrozzo M. Management of oral lichen planus. Am J Clin Dermatol. 2000;1(5):287–306.
12. Heitz-Mayfield LJ. Peri-implant diseases: diagnosis and risk indicators. J Clin Periodontol. 2008;35(8 Suppl):292–304.
13. Karbach J, Callaway A, Kwon YD, d'Hoedt B, Al-Nawas B. Comparison of five parameters as risk factors for peri-mucositis. Int J Oral Maxillofac Implants. 2009;24(3):491–6.
14. Roos-Jansaker AM, Renvert H, Lindahl C, Renvert S. Nine- to fourteen-year follow-up of implant treatment. Part III: factors associated with peri-implant lesions. J Clin Periodontol. 2006;33(4):296–301.
15. Ferreira SD, Silva GL, Cortelli JR, Costa JE, Costa FO. Prevalence and risk variables for peri-implant disease in Brazilian subjects. J Clin Periodontol. 2006;33(12):929–35.
16. Ferreira CF, Buttendorf AR, de Souza JG, Dalago H, Guenther SF, Bianchini MA. Prevalence of peri-implant diseases: analyses of associated factors. Eur J Prosthodont Restor Dent. 2015;23(4):199–206.
17. Heitz-Mayfield LJA, Salvi GE. Peri-implant mucositis. J Periodontol. 2018;89(Suppl 1):S257–S66.
18. Schwarz F, Derks J, Monje A, Wang HL. Peri-implantitis. J Clin Periodontol. 2018;45(Suppl 20):S246–S66.
19. Figuero E, Graziani F, Sanz I, Herrera D, Sanz M. Management of peri-implant mucositis and peri-implantitis. Periodontol 2000. 2014;66(1):255–73.
20. Renvert S, Polyzois I, Maguire R. Re-osseointegration on previously contaminated surfaces: a systematic review. Clin Oral Implants Res. 2009;20(Suppl 4):216–27.
21. Renvert S, Aghazadeh A, Hallstrom H, Persson GR. Factors related to peri-implantitis—a retrospective study. Clin Oral Implants Res. 2014;25(4):522–9.

22. Alqahtani F, Alqahtani M, Shafqat SS, Akram Z, Al-Kheraif AA, Javed F. Efficacy of mechanical debridement with adjunctive probiotic therapy in the treatment of peri-implant mucositis in cigarette-smokers and never-smokers. Clin Implant Dent Relat Res. 2019;21(4):734–40.
23. Alqahtani F, Alqhtani N, Alkhtani F, Divakar DD, Al-Kheraif AA, Javed F. Efficacy of mechanical debridement with and without adjunct antimicrobial photodynamic therapy in the treatment of peri-implantitis among moderate cigarette-smokers and waterpipe-users. Photodiagn Photodyn Ther. 2019;28:153–8.
24. Javed F, BinShabaib MS, Alharthi SS, Qadri T. Role of mechanical curettage with and without adjunct antimicrobial photodynamic therapy in the treatment of peri-implant mucositis in cigarette smokers: a randomized controlled clinical trial. Photodiagn Photodyn Ther. 2017;18:331–4.
25. Romanos GE, Javed F, Delgado-Ruiz RA, Calvo-Guirado JL. Peri-implant diseases: a review of treatment interventions. Dent Clin N Am. 2015;59(1):157–78.
26. Javed F, Romanos GE. Does photodynamic therapy enhance standard antibacterial therapy in dentistry? Photomed Laser Surg. 2013;31(11):512–8.
27. Javed F, Al Amri MD, Kellesarian SV, Al-Askar M, Al-Kheraif AA, Romanos GE. Laminin coatings on implant surfaces promote osseointegration: fact or fiction? Arch Oral Biol. 2016;68:153–61.
28. Ahmed P, Bukhari IA, Albaijan R, Sheikh SA, Vohra F. The effectiveness of photodynamic and antibiotic gel therapy as an adjunct to mechanical debridement in the treatment of peri-implantitis among diabetic patients. Photodiagn Photodyn Ther. 2020;32:102077.
29. Albaker AM, ArRejaie AS, Alrabiah M, Abduljabbar T. Effect of photodynamic and laser therapy in the treatment of peri-implant mucositis: a systematic review. Photodiagn Photodyn Ther. 2018;21:147–52.
30. Chambrone L, Wang HL, Romanos GE. Antimicrobial photodynamic therapy for the treatment of periodontitis and peri-implantitis: an American Academy of periodontology best evidence review. J Periodontol. 2018;89(7):783–803.
31. Romeo U, Nardi GM, Libotte F, Sabatini S, Palaia G, Grassi FR. The antimicrobial photodynamic therapy in the treatment of peri-implantitis. Int J Dent. 2016;2016:7692387.
32. van Winkelhoff AJ. Antibiotics in the treatment of peri-implantitis. Eur J Oral Implantol. 2012;5(Suppl):S43–50.
33. Al Hamoudi N. Is antimicrobial photodynamic therapy an effective treatment for chronic periodontitis in diabetes mellitus and cigarette smokers: a systematic review and meta-analysis. Photodiagn Photodyn Ther. 2017;19:375–82.
34. Al Hafez ASS, Ingle N, Alshayeb AA, Tashery HM, Alqarni AAM, Alshamrani SH. Effectiveness of mechanical debridement with and without adjunct antimicrobial photodynamic for treating peri-implant mucositis among prediabetic cigarette-smokers and non-smokers. Photodiagn Photodyn Ther. 2020;31:101912.
35. Adell R, Lekholm U, Rockler B, Branemark PI, Lindhe J, Eriksson B, et al. Marginal tissue reactions at osseointegrated titanium fixtures (I). A 3-year longitudinal prospective study. Int J Oral Maxillofac Surg. 1986;15(1):39–52.
36. Zarb GA, Schmitt A. The longitudinal clinical effectiveness of osseointegrated dental implants: the Toronto study. Part III: problems and complications encountered. J Prosthet Dent. 1990;64(2):185–94.
37. Marquez IC. The role of keratinized tissue and attached gingiva in maintaining periodontal/peri-implant health. Gen Dent. 2004;52(1):74–8; quiz 9.
38. Kim BS, Kim YK, Yun PY, Yi YJ, Lee HJ, Kim SG, et al. Evaluation of peri-implant tissue response according to the presence of keratinized mucosa. Oral Surg Oral Med Oral Pathol Oral Radiol Endod. 2009;107(3):e24–8.
39. Bouri A Jr, Bissada N, Al-Zahrani MS, Faddoul F, Nouneh I. Width of keratinized gingiva and the health status of the supporting tissues around dental implants. Int J Oral Maxillofac Implants. 2008;23(2):323–6.

40. Lang NP, Mombelli A, Tonetti MS, Bragger U, Hammerle CH. Clinical trials on therapies for peri-implant infections. Ann Periodontol. 1997;2(1):343–56.
41. Persson LG, Ericsson I, Berglundh T, Lindhe J. Guided bone regeneration in the treatment of periimplantitis. Clin Oral Implants Res. 1996;7(4):366–72.
42. Ericsson I, Persson LG, Berglundh T, Edlund T, Lindhe J. The effect of antimicrobial therapy on periimplantitis lesions. An experimental study in the dog. Clin Oral Implants Res. 1996;7(4):320–8.
43. Froum SJ, Froum SH, Rosen PS. A regenerative approach to the successful treatment of Peri-implantitis: a consecutive series of 170 implants in 100 patients with 2- to 10-year follow-up. Int J Periodontics Restorative Dent. 2015;35(6):857–63.
44. Roy M, Loutan L, Garavaglia G, Hashim D. Removal of osseointegrated dental implants: a systematic review of explantation techniques. Clin Oral Investig. 2020;24(1):47–60.
45. Zitzmann NU, Berglundh T. Definition and prevalence of peri-implant diseases. J Clin Periodontol. 2008;35(8 Suppl):286–91.
46. Lindhe J, Meyle J, Group DoEWoP. Peri-implant diseases: consensus report of the sixth European workshop on periodontology. J Clin Periodontol. 2008;35(8 Suppl):282–5.
47. Dixon DR, London RM. Restorative design and associated risks for peri-implant diseases. Periodontol 2000. 2019;81(1):167–78.
48. Korsch M, Walther W, Bartols A. Cement-associated peri-implant mucositis. A 1-year follow-up after excess cement removal on the peri-implant tissue of dental implants. Clin Implant Dent Relat Res. 2017;19(3):523–9.
49. Yue ZG, Zhang HD, Yang JW, Hou JX. Comparison of residual cement between CAD/CAM customized abutments and stock abutments via digital measurement in vitro. Beijing Da Xue Xue Bao. 2020;53(1):69–75.
50. Thoma DS, Naenni N, Figuero E, Hammerle CHF, Schwarz F, Jung RE, et al. Effects of soft tissue augmentation procedures on peri-implant health or disease: a systematic review and meta-analysis. Clin Oral Implants Res. 2018;29(Suppl 15):32–49.
51. Heitz-Mayfield LJA, Salvi GE, Mombelli A, Loup PJ, Heitz F, Kruger E, et al. Supportive peri-implant therapy following anti-infective surgical peri-implantitis treatment: 5-year survival and success. Clin Oral Implants Res. 2018;29(1):1–6.
52. Costa FO, Takenaka-Martinez S, Cota LO, Ferreira SD, Silva GL, Costa JE. Peri-implant disease in subjects with and without preventive maintenance: a 5-year follow-up. J Clin Periodontol. 2012;39(2):173–81.
53. Olmedo DG, Paparella ML, Brandizzi D, Cabrini RL. Reactive lesions of peri-implant mucosa associated with titanium dental implants: a report of 2 cases. Int J Oral Maxillofac Surg. 2010;39(5):503–7.
54. Buchner A, Shnaiderman-Shapiro A, Vered M. Relative frequency of localized reactive hyperplastic lesions of the gingiva: a retrospective study of 1675 cases from Israel. J Oral Pathol Med. 2010;39(8):631–8.
55. Al-Khateeb TH. Benign oral masses in a northern Jordanian population-a retrospective study. Open Dent J. 2009;3:147–53.
56. Dojcinovic I, Richter M, Lombardi T. Occurrence of a pyogenic granuloma in relation to a dental implant. J Oral Maxillofac Surg. 2010;68(8):1874–6.
57. Etoz OA, Soylu E, Kilic K, Gunhan O, Akcay H, Alkan A. A reactive lesion (pyogenic granuloma) associated with dental implant: a case report. J Oral Implantol. 2013;39(6):733–6.
58. Gorpas D, Davari P, Bec J, Fung MA, Marcu L, Farwell DG, et al. Time-resolved fluorescence spectroscopy for the diagnosis of oral lichen planus. Clin Exp Dermatol. 2018;43(5):546–52.
59. Nosratzehi T. Oral lichen planus: an overview of potential risk factors, biomarkers and treatments. Asian Pac J Cancer Prev. 2018;19(5):1161–7.
60. Anitua E, Pinas L, Escuer-Artero V, Fernandez RS, Alkhraisat MH. Short dental implants in patients with oral lichen planus: a long-term follow-up. Br J Oral Maxillofac Surg. 2018;56(3):216–20.
61. Thongprasom K. Oral lichen planus: challenge and management. Oral Dis. 2018;24(1–2):172–3.

62. Arduino PG, Campolongo MG, Sciannameo V, Conrotto D, Gambino A, Cabras M, et al. Randomized, placebo-controlled, double-blind trial of clobetasol propionate 0.05% in the treatment of oral lichen planus. Oral Dis. 2018;24(5):772–7.
63. Chiang CP, Yu-Fong Chang J, Wang YP, Wu YH, Lu SY, Sun A. Oral lichen planus—differential diagnoses, serum autoantibodies, hematinic deficiencies, and management. J Formos Med Assoc. 2018;117(9):756–65.
64. Agha-Hosseini F, Rohani B. Evaluation of the effects of dental implants on oral lesions. J Contemp Dent Pract. 2015;16(5):400–6.
65. Pons-Fuster A, Jornet PL. Dental implants in patients with oral lichen planus: a narrative review. Quintessence Int. 2014;45(7):599–603.
66. Petruzzi M, De Benedittis M, Cortelazzi R, Milillo L, Lucchese A, Serpico R, et al. Implant rehabilitation in patients with oral lichen planus: an overview. Clin Oral Investig. 2012;16(5):1347–52.
67. Mostafa B, Zakaria M. Evaluation of combined topical ozone and steroid therapy in management of oral lichen planus. Open Access Maced J Med Sci. 2018;6(5):879–84.
68. Hoseinpour Jajarm H, Asadi R, Bardideh E, Shafaee H, Khazaei Y, Emadzadeh M. The effects of photodynamic and low-level laser therapy for treatment of oral lichen planus-a systematic review and meta-analysis. Photodiagn Photodyn Ther. 2018;23:254–60.
69. Scully C, Carrozzo M. Oral mucosal disease: lichen planus. Br J Oral Maxillofac Surg. 2008;46(1):15–21.
70. Aboushelib MN, Elsafi MH. Clinical management protocol for dental implants inserted in patients with active lichen planus. J Prosthodont. 2017;26(1):29–33.

Prosthetic Role in Peri-Implant Soft Tissue Management: Treatment Planning Phase

7

Mohamed Moataz Khamis

7.1 Introduction

Loss of teeth is always associated with loss of alveolar bone and soft tissue. Functional and esthetic restoration of missing teeth necessitates not only tooth restoration (white esthetics) but restoration of lost bone and soft tissue (pink esthetics). Despite the different prosthetic options, dental implants are currently among the best to restore missing teeth because of the many advantages they provide.

Dental implant treatment involves the coordination of a team of multiple specialists, including prosthodontists, periodontists, surgeons, and dental technicians. Prosthodontists are supposedly the first of the team members to meet and select proper candidates from those who seek prosthetic restoration of their missing teeth. They should be able, through a well-organized treatment plan, to determine, together with the help of the other team members, the potential candidates for a successful implant treatment.

The demand for esthetic implant restorations raises the question of whether the final esthetic result is totally dependent on prosthetic procedures or whether there is a need for surgical intervention and reconstruction. An additional concern is how far can prosthetics contribute to peri-implant soft tissue management and esthetics.

Tooth restoration or white esthetics can totally be achieved by prosthetic techniques and procedures through the construction of a restoration having proper tooth shape, shade, size, position, and alignment. However, soft tissue or pink esthetics can be achieved by a combination of surgical and prosthetic techniques. The surgical role involves proper implant positioning, together with bone and soft tissue augmentation and management. In contrast, the prosthetic role involves many steps that have a direct impact on the final soft tissue outcome.

M. M. Khamis (✉)
Department of Prosthodontics, Faculty of Dentistry, Alexandria University, Alexandria, Egypt

M. Hassan (ed.), *Peri-Implant Soft Tissue Management*,
https://doi.org/10.1007/978-3-031-45516-2_7

Although the surgical role is the main player in soft tissue reconstruction and management, prosthetics can sometimes solve problems that are difficult to manage surgically and can augment the surgical procedures to reach satisfactory results. It is therefore imperative to highlight how prosthetics can contribute to soft tissue management and health around implants to promote an effective collaboration between the different specialty team members.

7.2 Patient Selection

The first step in implant treatment is the proper selection of potentially successful candidates for implant restorations. Although the first specialty to choose potential candidates are usually prosthodontists, a consultation with the surgeon and/or periodontist is highly recommended, especially if peri-implant soft tissue management is necessary. Patient selection involves many considerations involving prosthetic, surgical, psychological, and financial issues. However, regarding soft tissue management, specific points should be considered.

7.2.1 Amount of Soft Tissue Showing During Smiling

Restoring peri-implant hard and soft tissues can be performed for functional and/or esthetic reasons. In the esthetic zone, the amount of soft tissue showing during smiling determines whether treatment planning should be geared toward a functional or esthetic protocol. In the case of an esthetic protocol, a combination of surgical and prosthetic approaches should be implemented.

According to Johnson [1], alveolar bone resorbs and loses about 25% of its volume during the first year and up to 40–60% in width within the first 3 years of tooth loss. Schropp et al. [2] reported that as much as 40% to 50% of alveolar width and 20% to 30% of height are irreversibly lost during the first year following extraction. Most of the dimensional alterations of the alveolar ridge, whether horizontal or vertical, take place during the first 3 months of healing [3]. This implies that patients seeking tooth restoration, especially those with a high smile line in the esthetic zone following a few months of tooth extraction, would likely require both surgical (bone and/or soft tissue grafting) and prosthetic approaches (Fig. 7.1).

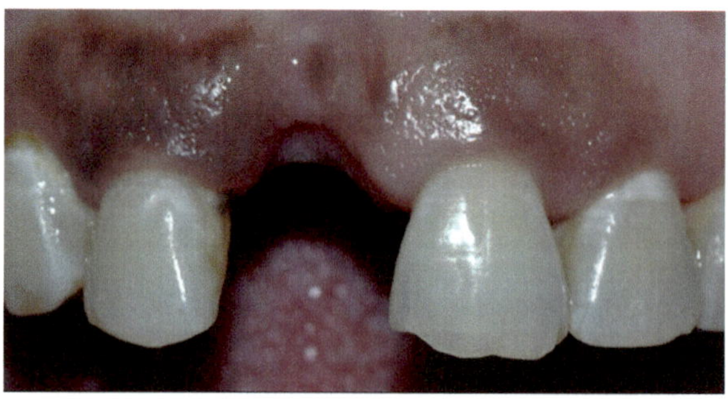

Fig. 7.1 Soft tissue defect requiring surgical and prosthetic approaches for correction

7.2.2 Understanding Patient Demands and Expectations

Understanding patient expectations of the final prosthetic result, especially the esthetic part, is sometimes a difficult task. Lack of consideration of patient expectations might result in an unsatisfied patient.

In patients with low lip lines or when soft tissues do not show during smiling, treatment planning is usually directed toward functionally restoring teeth, concentrating on white esthetics, and not necessarily restoring pink esthetics if their deficiency is not compromising functional implant positioning. Restoring conditions with bone and soft tissue defects without augmentation usually results in restorations that are longer occluso-cervically than their neighboring counterparts. In most of the cases, this does not cause an esthetic problem as it does not show during smiling (Fig. 7.2a, b). Adding a pink-colored section to the restoration (commonly gingival porcelain) can sometimes be used to improve the esthetic outcome (Fig. 7.3). However, it is important to understand the patient's demands and expectations. Even though they do not show during smiling, some patients still psychologically prefer bone and soft tissue augmentation to naturally restore their soft tissue defects (Fig. 7.4). This must be clear from the start to tailor the treatment plan accordingly.

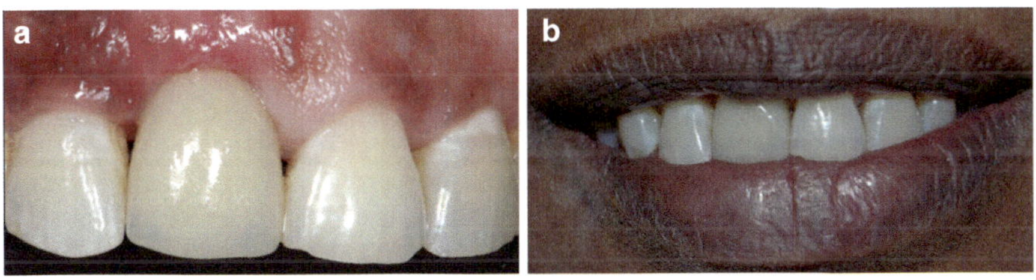

Fig. 7.2 (**a**) Long restoration occluso-cervically due to lack of augmentation of bone and soft tissue defect. (**b**) Acceptable esthetic result because of the low lip line

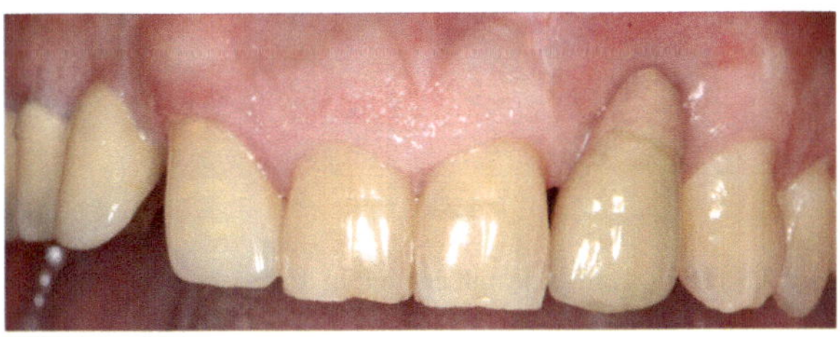

Fig. 7.3 Adding gingival porcelain of suitable shade to improve the esthetic outcome

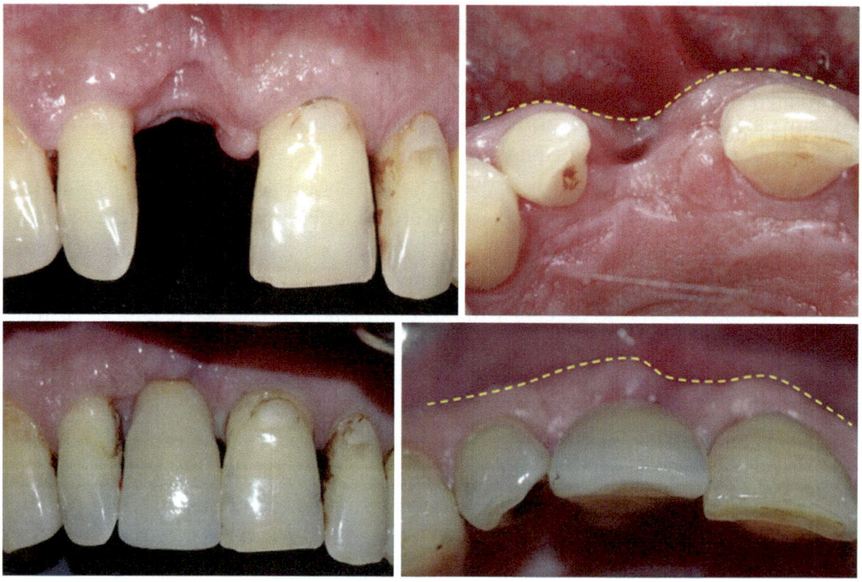

Fig. 7.4 Bone and soft tissue defect requiring a staged grafting procedure. Acceptable prosthetic result following a staged guided bone regeneration procedure

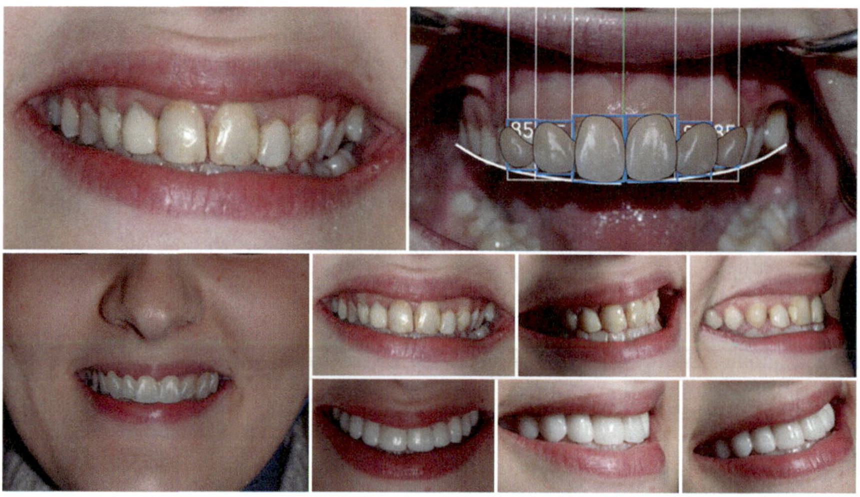

Fig. 7.5 Digital smile design can aid in understanding patient expectations

7.2.3 Digital Smile Design

One way of understanding patient expectations is through a digital smile design [4–6], which can be used to fabricate a mockup. This way, an objective decision can be reached based on patient acceptance of the result (Fig. 7.5). After patient approval, the digital smile design can be used to fabricate a surgical guide for proper implant placement and soft tissue augmentation. It can also be used to construct a temporary restoration [5, 6].

7.3 Treatment Planning

Once an appropriate patient is selected, treatment planning should be performed. Treatment planning involves many considerations, including implant selection, placement techniques, biomechanics, soft tissue management, and prosthetic procedures, all geared the placement of the implant in a proper prosthetic position to reach a final acceptable result. Knowing the capabilities of the team members of different specialties is important to be able to coordinate the efforts to reach optimal results.

7.3.1 Esthetic Implant Positioning

The demand for an esthetic implant restoration is always increasing. Patient demands and expectations when implants are used to restore missing teeth are usually very high and in some cases unrealistic. However, to achieve ultimate esthetic results, some considerations need to be addressed, including proper patient selection, implant positioning and alignment, creation of a proper emergence profile, and restoring lost bone and soft tissue.

To achieve an acceptable, esthetic peri-implant soft tissue contour, implants should be properly positioned and aligned in three dimensions: mesiodistally, labiolingually, and apicoincisally. In the esthetic zone, implants should be used to restore missing teeth only if they can be placed in a proper prosthetic position or else it would be difficult to combine esthetics together with a hygienic design. To ensure proper positioning and alignment as treatment planned, surgical guides can be fabricated and used.

According to the degree of limitation of the surgical guide, guides can be nonlimiting, partially limiting, or completely limiting [7]. Conventional surgical guides are usually nonlimiting. They are mainly intended to guide implant placement from a prosthetic point of view but do not ensure accurate positioning or limit the depth of drilling (Fig. 7.6). They usually guide implant direction. CAD-CAM fabricated guides can be partially or completely limiting. Partially limiting guides control the direction and depth of drilling for the first few drills. The final drill, however, is used free hand guided by the direction of the previous drills (Fig. 7.7). The completely limiting guides control the drilling procedure from the start all the way to implant placement. They therefore guide implant placement prosthetically and surgically as implant depth and relation to important anatomical structures are also controlled [5, 7] (Fig. 7.8).

Studies comparing the accuracy of implant placement between partially and fully guided CAD-CAM fabricated surgical guides do not show a clinically

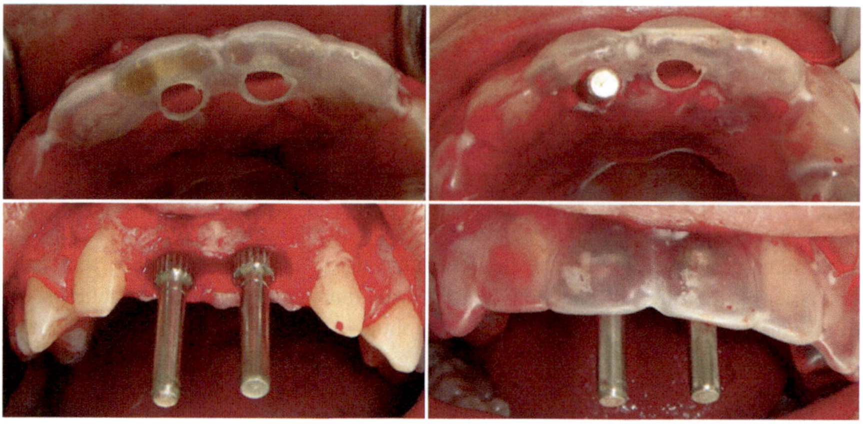

Fig. 7.6 Nonlimiting conventional surgical guide

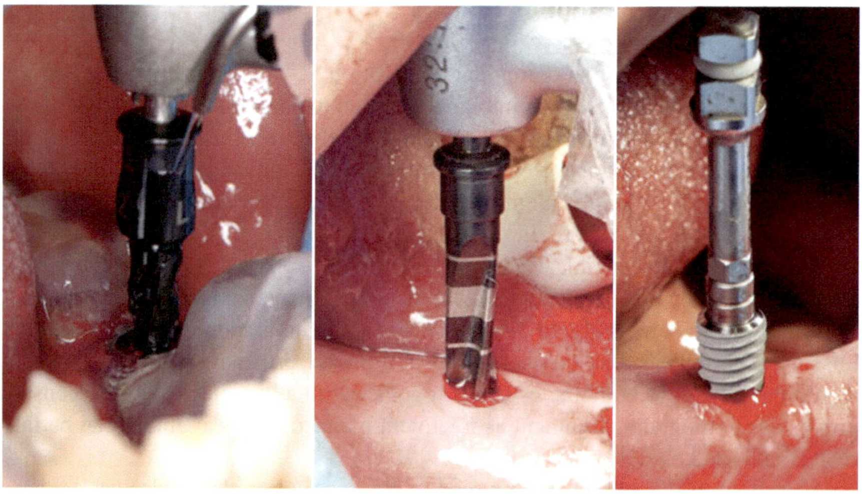

Fig. 7.7 Partially limiting guide

significant difference between both techniques [8]. However, one of the concerns of using those guides was the difficulty of the cooling solution to reach the osteotomy site during drilling because of the precision between the drill shank and the guiding holes of the surgical guide. The inability to provide sufficient irrigation during drilling might compromise the peri-implant hard and soft tissues. To improve the efficiency of irrigation and at the same time maintain guidance, C-shaped guide holes can be used (Fig. 7.9). In a study comparing the peri-implant soft and hard tissues

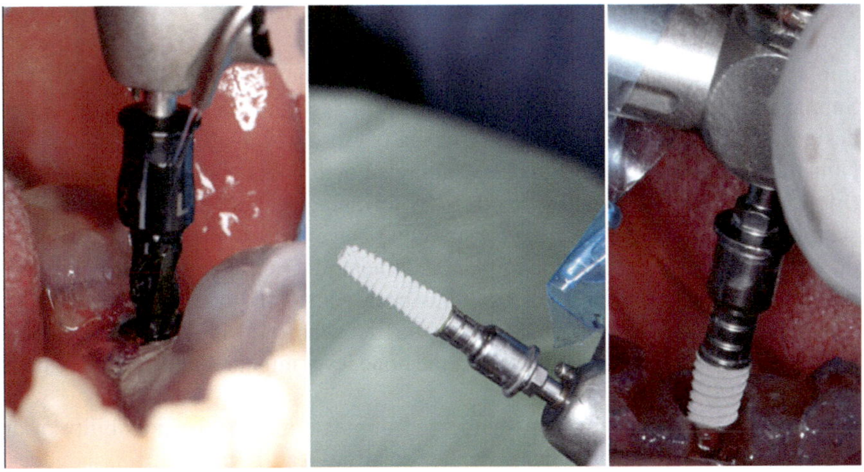

Fig. 7.8 Completely limiting guide

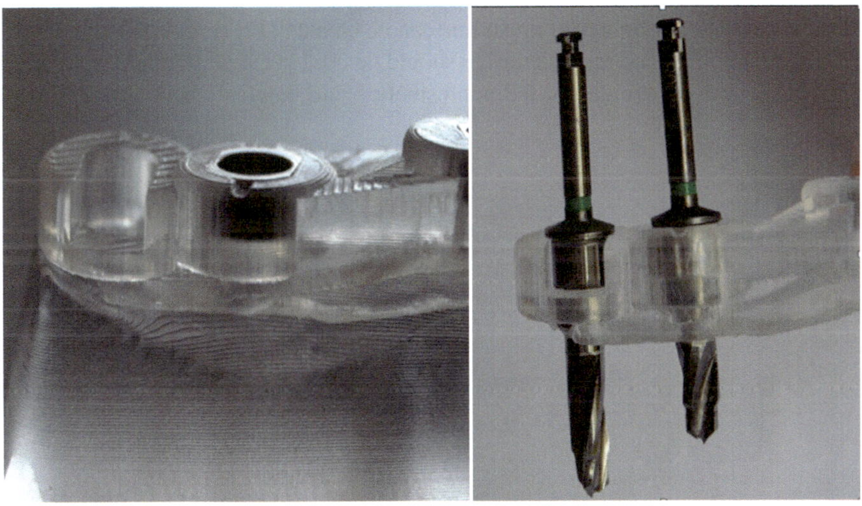

Fig. 7.9 C-shaped guide holes

after flapless implant placement by using fully guided versus partially guided surgical guides with cylindrical versus C-shaped guide holes, no clinical or radiographic difference was found [9]. Implants can therefore be placed accurately by using CAD-CAM fabricated guides without compromising peri-implant hard and soft tissues [10, 11].

7.3.2 Submerged Versus Non-submerged Implants

Implants can be placed by using a submerged or a non-submerged protocol [12]. Submerged implants can have a short 1 mm or less smooth collar height. Some designs do not have a smooth collar, especially those with platform switching [13]. Non-submerged implant designs have a long smooth collar about 2.5 mm in length (Fig. 7.10). Those implants provide two advantages: first, they are kept non-submerged, eliminating the need for a second-stage surgery procedure with all its drawbacks; second, keeping the implant abutment junction (micro gap) supragingival. The implant abutment micro gap has been considered one of the reasons for crestal bone resorption that occurs during the first year following implant placement [14]. Keeping the micro gap away from the bone level might reduce the rate of bone resorption [15, 16].

The drawbacks of using non-submerged implants include the possibility of an unesthetic intraoral metal collar show, especially if peri-implant soft tissue recession occurs (Fig. 7.11). One way to overcome this problem is to use a submerged implant design together with a healing abutment placed at the time of implant insertion. This way, a second-stage procedure is avoided and at the same time a final restoration with a subgingival finish line can be created [12] (Fig. 7.12).

The non-submerged implant design should be used in cases when a second-stage procedure is to be avoided in the non-esthetic zone, implants have good primary

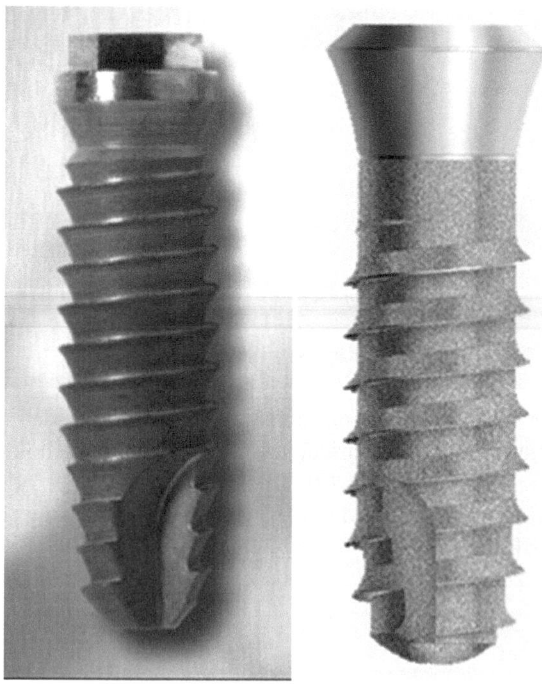

Fig. 7.10 Submerged implant design on the left. Non-submerged implant design on the right

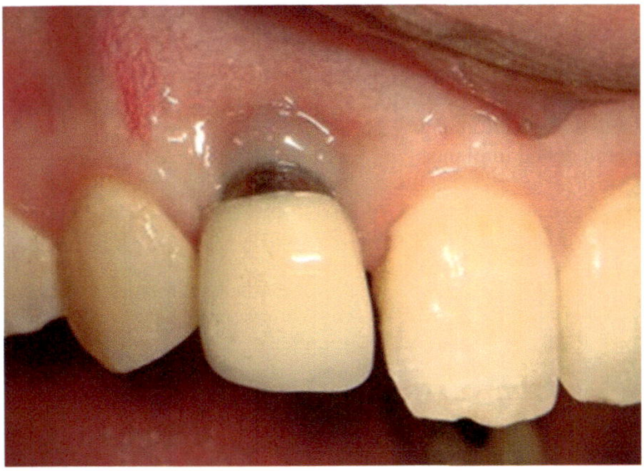

Fig. 7.11 Unesthetic metal collar show as a result of peri-implant soft tissue recession

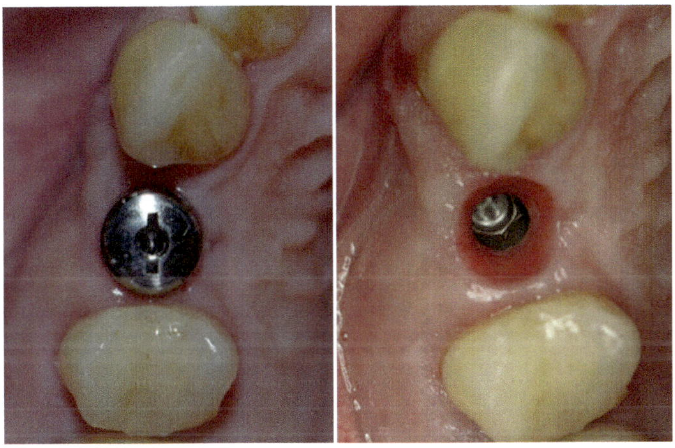

Fig. 7.12 Submerged implant design with a healing abutment attached at the time of implant placement, making it a single-stage procedure

stability, and preferably when there is no need for guided bone regeneration [12]. To overcome the unesthetic properties of single-stage implants, some companies provide implants with tooth-colored collars or implants totally made of zirconia [17].

7.4 Restoration Emergence Profile

The contour of the gingival margin of teeth is an important determinant of an esthetic smile. In spite of the difference in contour of the gingival margin among natural teeth, symmetry between contralateral teeth is essential to ensure uniformity. The contour of the gingival margin of teeth is determined by the facial bone contour, gingival texture, and emergence profile of the individual tooth [18]. The emergence profile of a tooth is its profile while emerging from the gingiva.

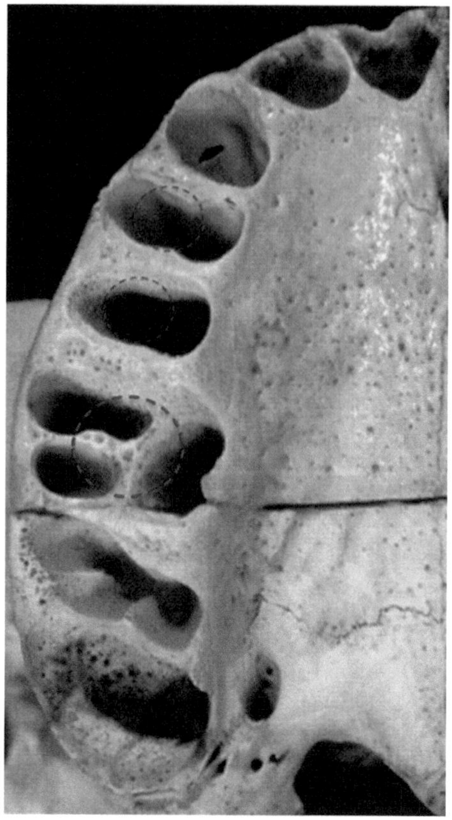

Fig. 7.13 Cross section of natural teeth at the bone level showing the difference between natural teeth cross section and round dental implants

The cross section of every tooth in the dental arch varies at the bone level (Fig. 7.13). The emergence profile and consequently the gingival margin contour therefore differ as they follow the configuration of the emergence profile of the tooth (Fig. 7.14). The cross section of maxillary incisors is usually triangular, canines are rhomboidal, premolars are oval, and molars are trapezoidal (Fig. 7.15).

When natural teeth are restored by using crowns, the emergence profile of the crown should be adjusted and designed to simulate the contralateral side, therefore maintaining a proper gingival margin contour. However, when dental implants are used, their cross section at the bone level is round which is different from all natural teeth that are never round (Fig. 7.16). If an implant restoration is designed with a round emergence profile, this will result in a gingival margin that is not symmetrical when compared to the natural contralateral tooth (Fig. 7.17). The clinician should be aware that the emergence profile of an implant restoration should change from round to triangular if an incisor is to be restored or oval if a premolar is to be restored and so on. This way, the gingival margin of the peri-implant mucosa can be properly and symmetrically contoured [19].

Changing the emergence profile of an implant restoration from round to oval should be performed within the distance between the bone level (implant platform)

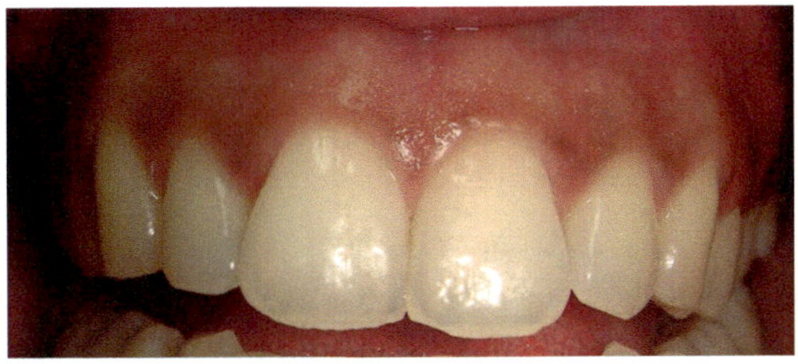

Fig. 7.14 Contour of the gingival margin of natural teeth varies from one tooth to another depending on the tooth emergence profile

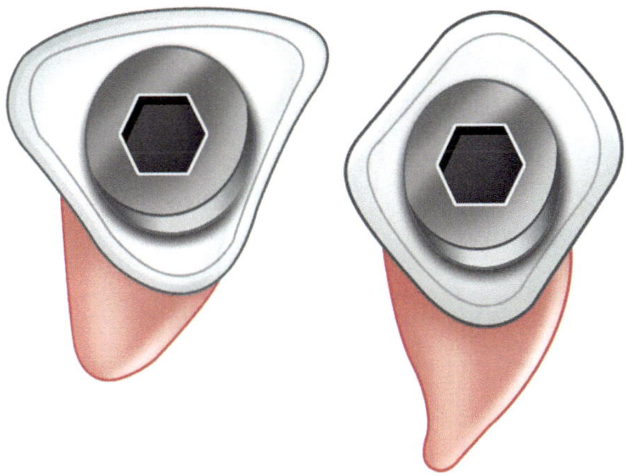

Fig. 7.15 Difference between the emergence profile of natural teeth and round dental implants

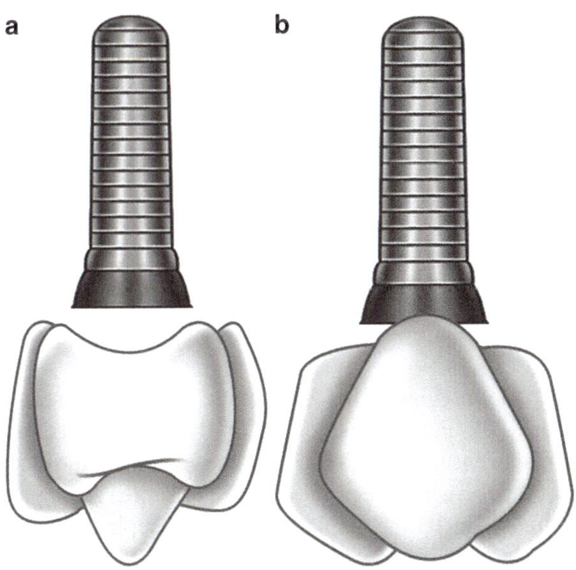

Fig. 7.16 The round implant cross section should be changed to the natural tooth emergence profile to restore the esthetic peri-implant soft tissue margin (**a**) proximal view. (**b**) facial view

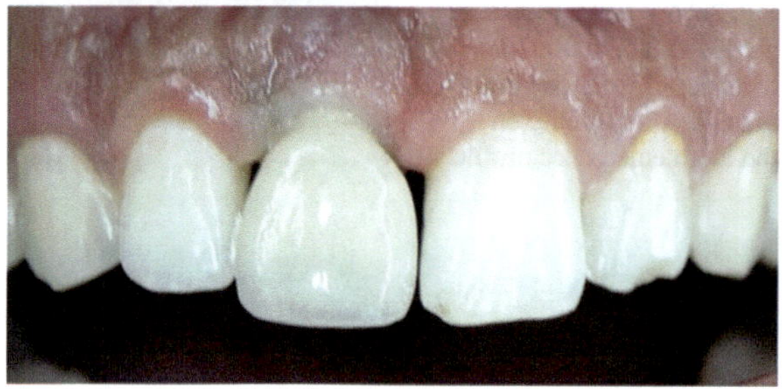

Fig. 7.17 Improperly designed transition between the round implant cross section and the triangular central incisor emergence profile compromising the overall esthetic result

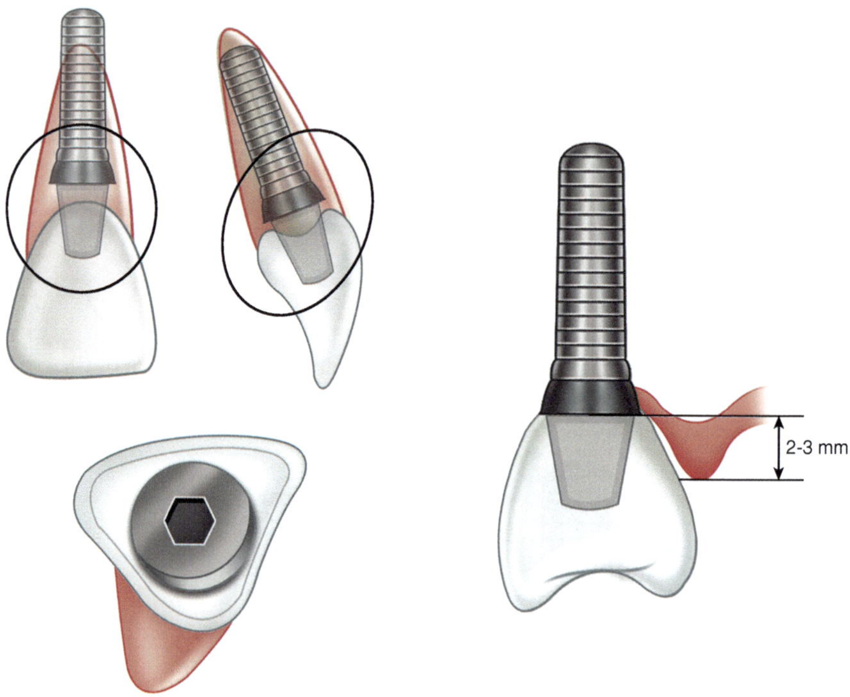

Fig. 7.18 Emergence profile change from round to triangular, oval, or rhomboidal should be performed within the distance between the implant platform and the peri-implant soft tissue margin

and the gingival margin (Fig. 7.18). An average of 3 mm is required to allow a smooth transition [20]. Proper positioning of the implant occluso-cervically is therefore important to ensure enough space for the creation of the emergence profile.

Creation of a proper emergence profile can be performed during most of the steps of implant treatment, including implant selection, implant positioning, flapless placement with a single-stage procedure, second-stage surgery, selection of a healing abutment, temporary crown fabrication, selection of an impression coping, abutment selection, and final prosthesis construction.

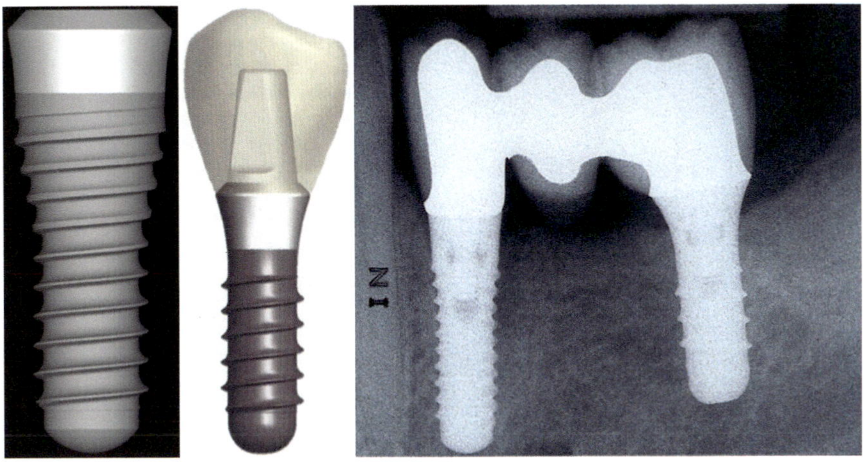

Fig. 7.19 Implants having a flared neck (collar) allow a smooth transition from implant to restoration

7.4.1 Implant Selection

Two features of an implant can affect the restoration emergence profile: the form of the implant neck portion and the implant platform diameter.

7.4.1.1 Form of the Neck Portion

Some implant designs have a flared implant collar (neck) (Fig. 7.19). Most of these implants are designed to be placed in a single-stage procedure. The flared implant neck allows a smooth transition from the implant to the restoration, resulting in a hygienic profile.

7.4.1.2 Implant Diameter

The selection of a proper implant diameter is essential to facilitate a proper emergence profile. An implant diameter that is slightly smaller than the diameter of the neck of a natural tooth (buccolingually and mesiodistally) allows a smooth transition between the implant platform and restoration (Fig. 7.20). An implant diameter that is too narrow makes it difficult to change from a round platform to a triangular or oval one. A sudden or abrupt change would be necessary, making it nonhygienic (Fig. 7.21). An alternative would be to emerge gradually, resulting in mesial and distal black triangles (Fig. 7.22). Too wide diameter is also unacceptable as it leads to an unesthetic restoration. Improper implant diameter selection will therefore result in loss of either esthetics or hygiene.

Choosing a narrow diameter is usually associated with reduced buccolingual diameter of the residual bone resulting from delayed restoration and bone resorption. In such cases, the ideal setting is to graft the bone, increasing its width to be able to choose the proper implant diameter. An alternative is to use an implant with a narrow diameter but a wide platform (Fig. 7.23).

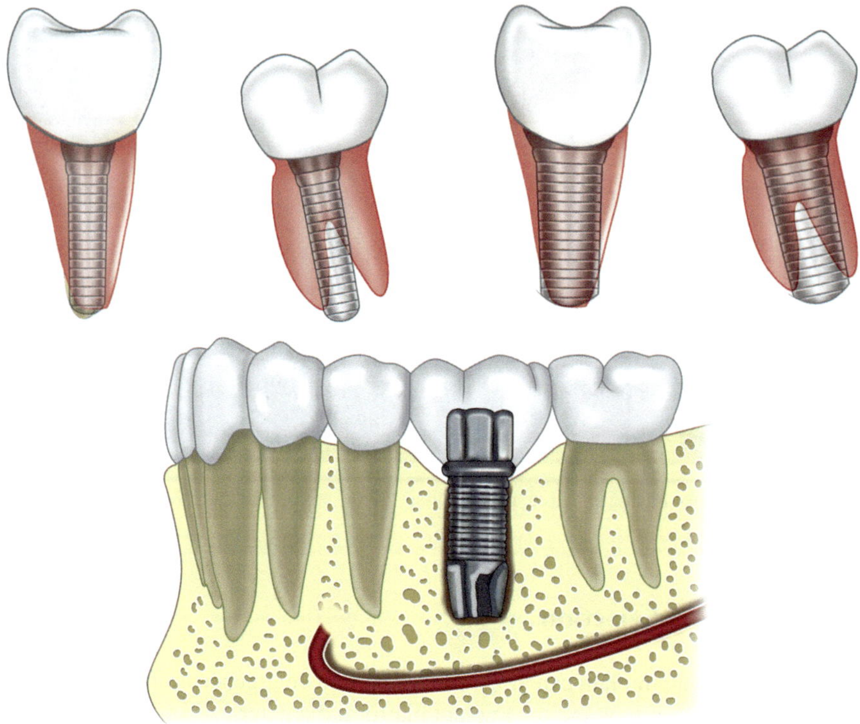

Fig. 7.20 Selection of a proper implant diameter ensures a proper emergence profile

Fig. 7.21 Too narrow implant diameter interfering with proper emergence profile

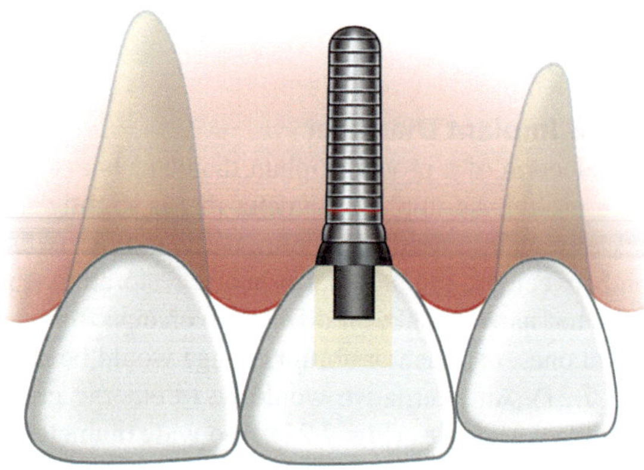

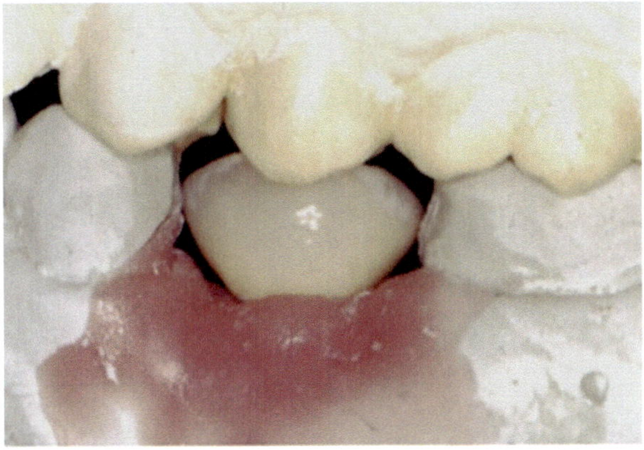

Fig. 7.22 Too narrow implant diameter resulting in an emergence profile with black mesial and distal triangles

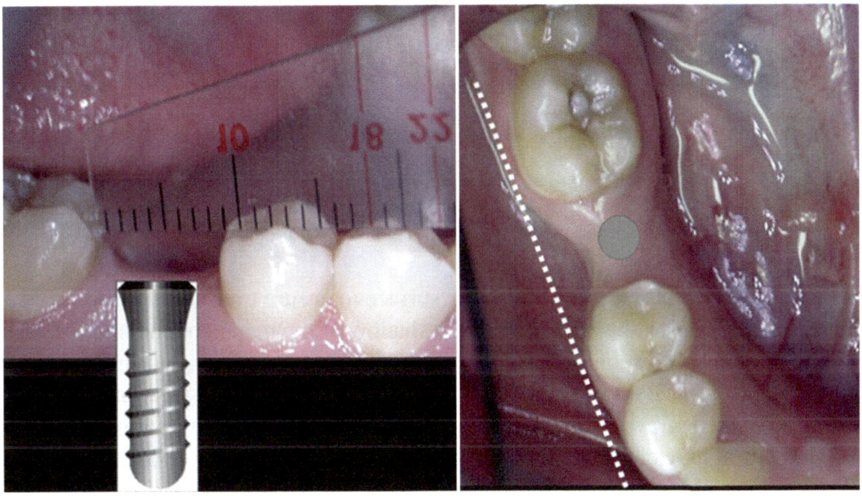

Fig. 7.23 An implant with a narrow diameter and a wide platform can be used in cases having a narrow buccolingual dimension and a wide mesiodistal one

7.4.2 Implant Positioning

The best position for an implant is the original tooth position provided that the tooth was in a proper position. An implant is positioned in three dimensions: mesiodistally, buccolingually, and apicoincisally.

7.4.2.1 Labio-Lingual Positioning

Maxillary and mandibular anterior implants should be positioned slightly palatal to the long axis of the tooth to be restored (Fig. 7.24). This is mainly to allow a

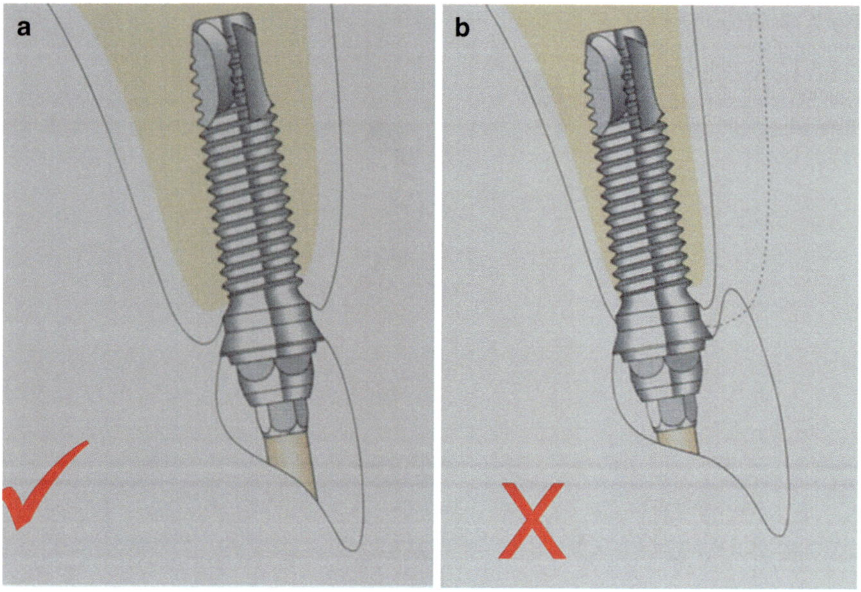

Fig. 7.24 (**a**) Long axis of maxillary and mandibular anterior teeth directed slightly palatal to allow the screw access channel to be located at the cingulum area. (**b**) Implant placed too far palatal, resulting in a short restoration that can be corrected by creating a lap ridge relation

thickness of the restoration on the labial surface to ensure translucency and avoid a thin weak restoration that might show the shadow of the metal abutment in the case of all ceramic restorations interfering with restoration esthetics by giving a grey hue. A slightly palatal position also allows a screw-retained restoration to have a palatally located screw access channel without the need for an angled abutment [20].

The problem exists in cases of delayed restoration after tooth extraction. Extensive labial bone resorption forces implant placement to be performed too far palatal, resulting in a short restoration (Figs. 7.25 and 7.26). To prosthetically correct this situation, a lap ridge relation can be designed to gingivally increase the length of the restoration (Fig. 7.24b) [20]. However, this ends up with an unhygienic emergence profile, resulting in peri-implant soft tissue problems. To avoid a palatal position, bone must be grafted to warrant a proper implant position. An alternative is to position the implant more apical to the ideal position, which should be 2–3 mm apical to the free gingival margin. Placing an implant 1 mm palatal to the idea position should be associated with a 1-mm apical position (Fig. 7.27).

Too far labial implant positioning results in a long restoration that cannot be easily corrected. A prosthetic solution would be to add a pink-colored restoration material (gingival porcelain) to the cervical part of the restoration (Fig. 7.28). This requires a talented technician to create an acceptable gingival contour and acceptable tissue shade of the gingival porcelain. In many cases, the implant is removed and a new one is placed in a proper position.

To avoid a lap ridge relation, the implant can be placed in an apical position.

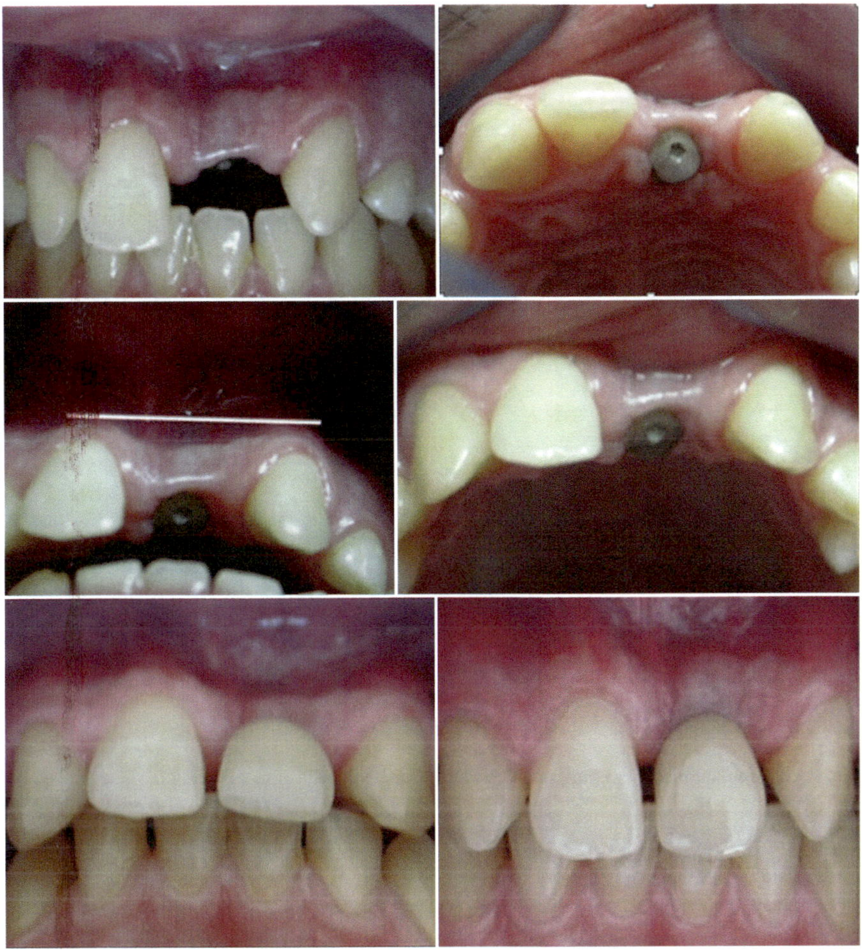

Fig. 7.25 Implant placed too far palatal resulting in a short restoration

7.4.2.2 Mesio-Distal Positioning

An implant should be positioned in the mesio-distal center of the tooth to be restored. Improper mesiodistal position results in compromised esthetics and/or hygiene (Fig. 7.29). An implant placed too close to a neighboring tooth will also prosthetically interfere with impression making, abutment attachment, and final restoration contour (Fig. 7.30).

When multiple implants are placed, proper mesiodistal implant orientation should be achieved bearing in mind the inter-implant distance as it has a direct effect on the configuration of the interdental papilla. An average distance of 3 mm is required between two adjacent implants to ensure acceptable interdental papilla configuration [21, 22] (Fig. 7.31).

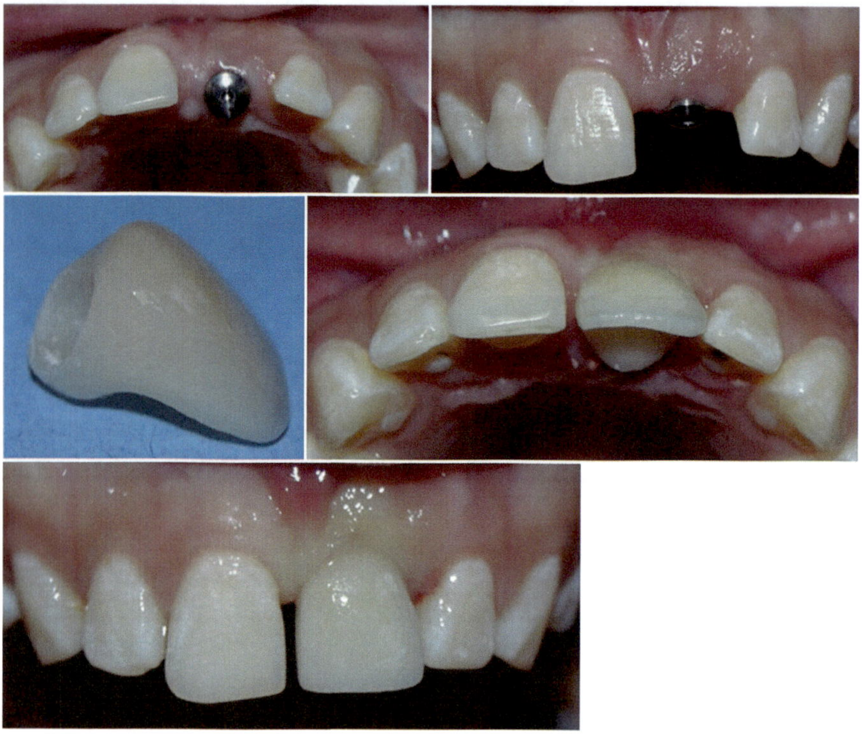

Fig. 7.26 Implant placed slightly palatal resulting in a slightly short restoration

Fig. 7.27 To avoid a lap ridge relation (**a**), implant can be placed in a more apical position (**b**)

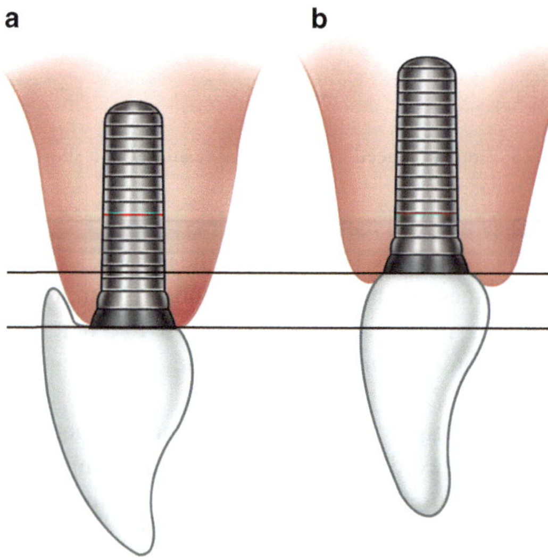

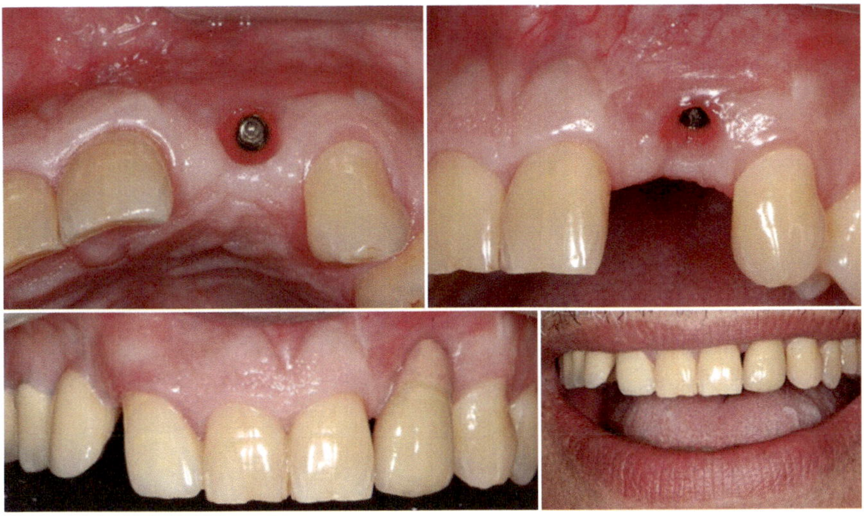

Fig. 7.28 Too far labial implant position results in a long restoration. Tissue-colored restorative material can improve the esthetic result

Fig. 7.29 Improper mesiodistal centralization of an implant compromises esthetics and hygiene

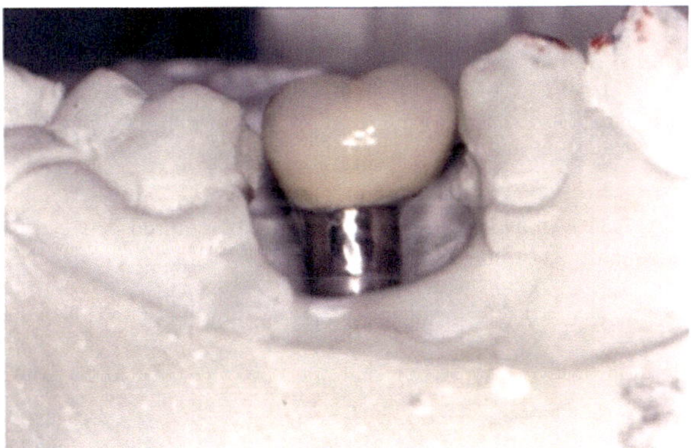

7.4.2.3 Apico-Incisal Positioning

In the esthetic zone, the ideal implant position should be submerged an average of 2–3 mm apical to the free gingival margin of neighboring teeth to be able to create an acceptable emergence profile (Fig. 7.32) [20]. Too deep apical implant position results in an unhygienic design, similar to a pocket in a natural tooth. Too far incisal positioning will not give a chance for a smooth transition between implant diameter and configuration and tooth design, resulting in a defective emergence profile together with the possibility of an abutment collar show compromising esthetics too.

A relation exists between implant diameter and its apico-incisal level of positioning. The more apical the implant position, the narrower the implant diameter to facilitate the creation of an acceptable emergence profile (Fig. 7.33).

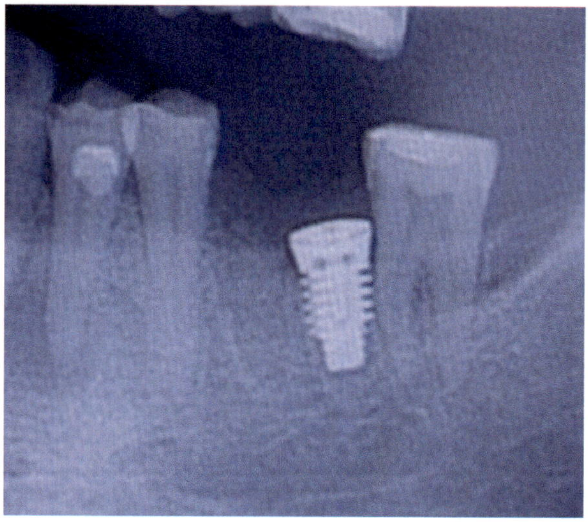

Fig. 7.30 Implant positioned too close to a neighboring tooth interfering with abutment and restoration attachment

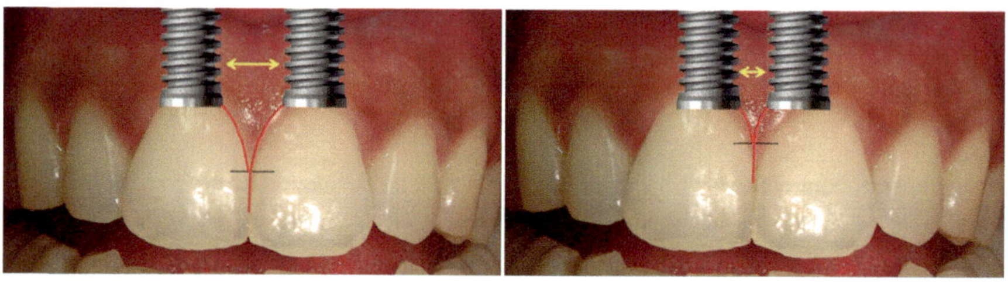

Fig. 7.31 An average distance of 3 mm is required between two adjacent implants to ensure an adequate size of interdental papilla

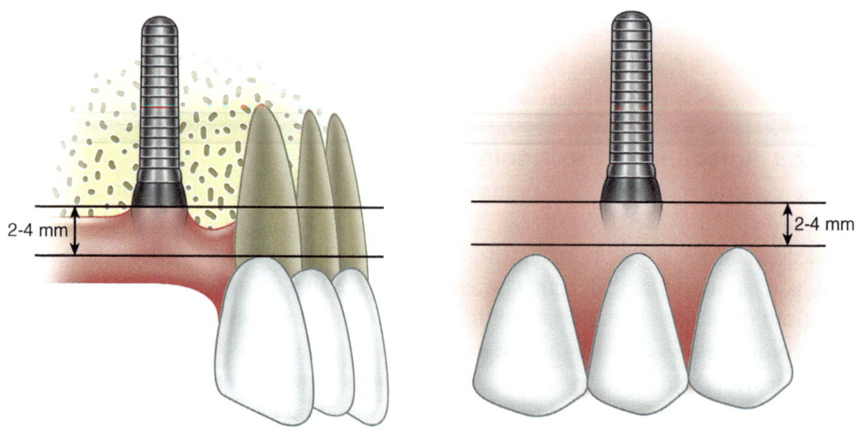

Fig. 7.32 A minimum space of 2–3 mm is required between the implant platform and free gingival margin to allow for a properly designed and contoured restoration emergence profile

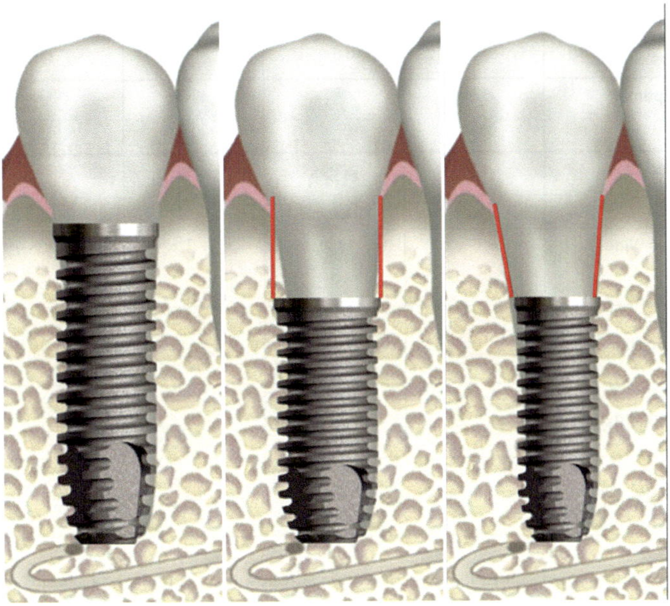

Fig. 7.33 The more apical the implant position, the narrower should be the implant diameter

Proper implant position in all three planes therefore has a direct effect on esthetics, biomechanics, phonetics, and hygiene [23–25]. If multiple implants are placed too close to each other, esthetics and hygiene would be compromised while biomechanics and phonetics would not be affected. If neighboring implants were placed too far from each other, esthetics, phonetics, and hygiene would be compromised, while biomechanics would not be affected (Fig. 7.34).

7.4.3 Immediate Implant Placement in a Freshly Extracted Socket by Using a Flapless Single-Stage Procedure

Preserving the gingiva, gingival margin, and interdental tissues around natural teeth following extraction is a goal that needs to be achieved. One way to do this is to extract the tooth atraumatically and place the implant flapless [26]. However, to preserve the soft tissue contour, a wide diameter stock healing abutment (Fig. 7.35) or a custom-made one (Fig. 7.36a,b) must be placed immediately at the time of implant placement. Creating a healing abutment with an identical emergence profile to the extracted tooth can aid the soft tissue to heal in a similar way to that around the natural tooth [27]. Multiple techniques are available for custom-made healing abutment fabrication [28, 29]. However, conventional methods require considerable chairside time. In addition, the intraorally polymerized resins used to construct the healing abutments have been reported to release byproducts and free monomers that have a detrimental effect on peri-implant tissues [30]. CAD-CAM technology can

Implant Position	Esthetics	Biomechanics	Phonetics	Hygiene
Optimal	Good	Good	Good	Good
Too Close	Great problems	Good	Good	Great problems
Too Wide	Great problems	Good	Difficult	Difficult
Too Angulated	Great problems	Difficult	Difficult	Difficult
Too Labial/Palatal	Difficult	Difficult	Difficult	Difficult

Good | Difficult | Great problems

Fig. 7.34 Relation between implant position and esthetics, biomechanics, phonetics, and hygiene

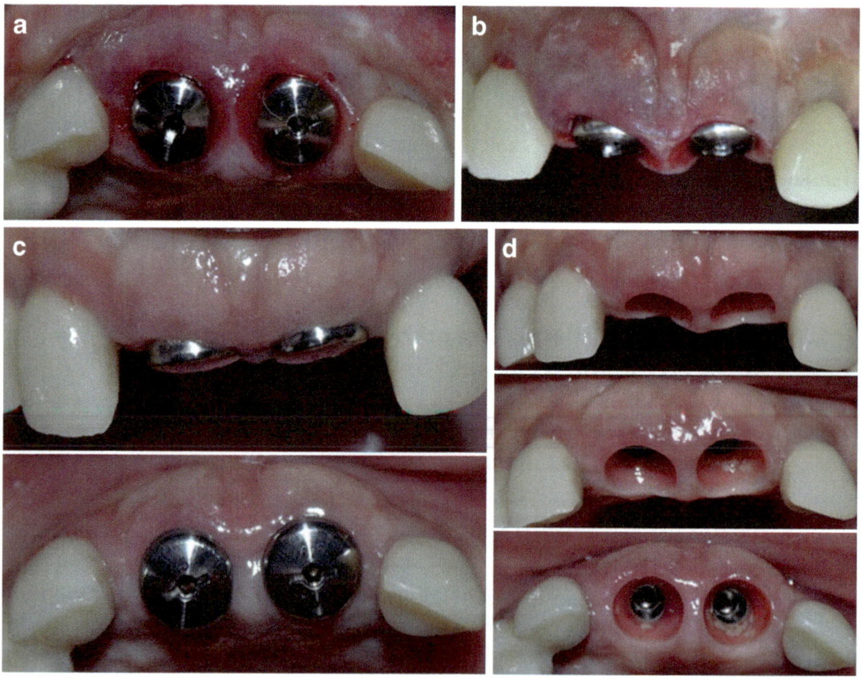

Fig. 7.35 (**a**, **b**) Stock healing abutment inserted immediately at the time of implant placement. (**c**, **d**) Soft tissue healing around stock healing abutments

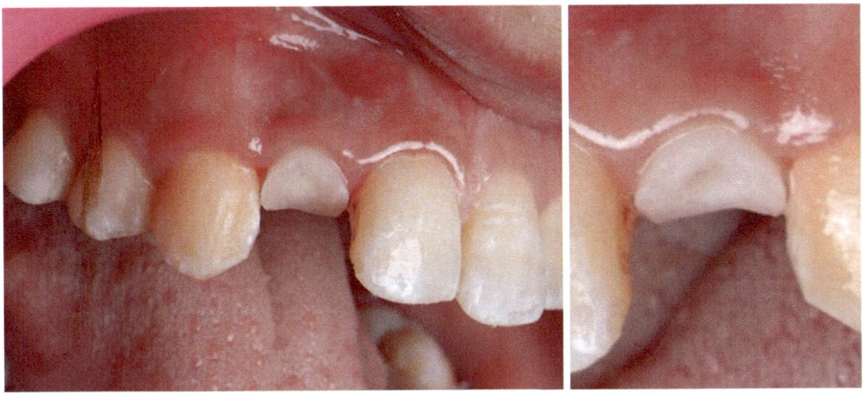

Fig. 7.36 Custom-made healing abutments attached to implants at the time of implant placement

nowadays aid in designing and fabrication of custom-made healing abutments. A custom-made healing abutment that duplicates the emergence profile of the tooth being extracted or the tooth on the contralateral side can be fabricated before extraction to be inserted immediately after implant placement [19] (Fig. 7.37a–h). The indirect fabrication avoids residual monomer and improves cell attachment. It also saves chairside time and ultimately patient satisfaction.

7.4.4 Second-Stage Surgery

Second-stage surgery can be performed by raising a flap and by using a tissue punch, lasers, and the cross technique. Raising a flap is usually indicated whenever the implant cannot be located or is covered by bone, as in cases of submerging the implant too much during insertion [31]. A tissue punch is a useful option in the non-esthetic zone. The drawback of which is that valuable keratinized soft tissue is lost (Fig. 7.38).

Dental lasers have improved dramatically in the past few years. By using a dental laser, peri-implant soft tissue can be carved to create an acceptable emergence profile [32, 33]. Again, lasers remove from the soft tissue, which might not be a wise decision in the esthetic zone. However, they can be a useful tool for refining peri-implant soft tissue contours and to perform hemostasis, especially if a direct digital impression is to be made [34–38] (Fig. 7.39).

To shape the peri-implant soft tissue contour, healing abutments can be placed at the second-stage surgery procedure. Custom-made healing abutments or temporary crowns can also be designed to create a favorable emergence profile that can be altered and modified by adjusting the healing abutment contour until a desirable shape is reached [19, 27]. The final restoration is made later on to duplicate the modified healing abutment.

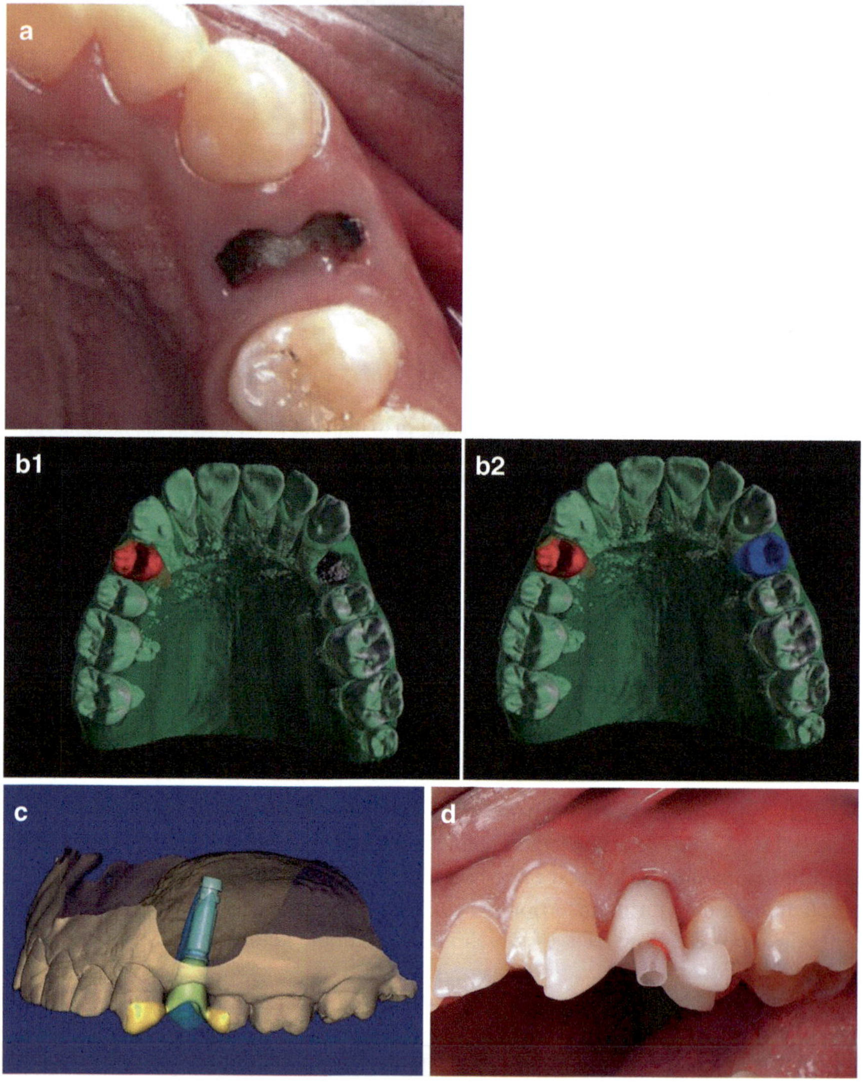

Fig. 7.37 (**a**) Non-restorable tooth, (**b1**) Segmented tooth (red) with maxillary cast aligned with DICOM file. (**b2**) Mirrored tooth (blue) in place. (**c**) Custom healing shell designed. (**d**) Clinical evaluation of custom healing shell with interim abutment in place. (**e**) Healing shell attached to the interim abutment. (**f**) Custom healing abutment in place. (**g**) Custom healing abutment out of occlusion. (**h**) Definitive restoration in place

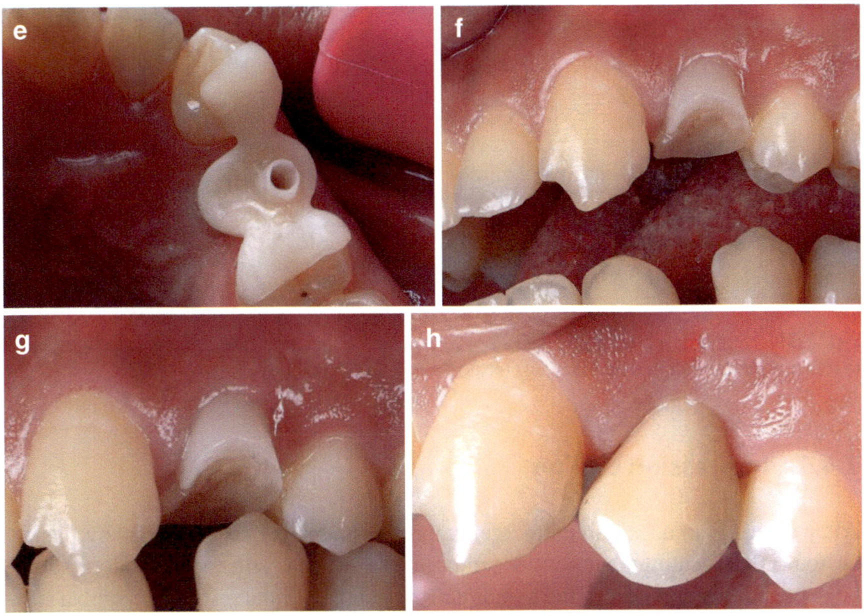

Fig. 7.37 (continued)

Fig. 7.38 Tissue punch is used to expose the implant during the second-stage surgery procedure

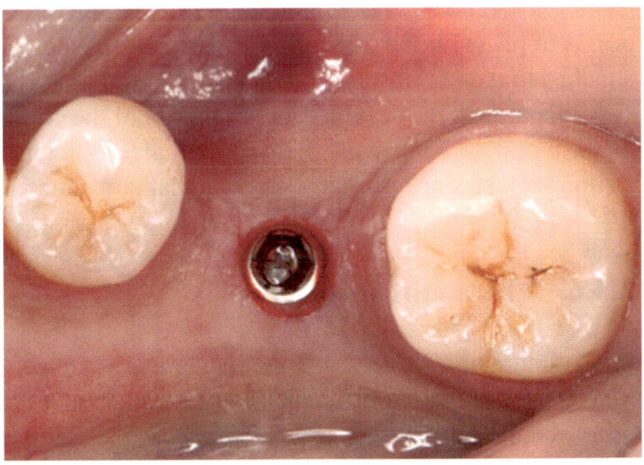

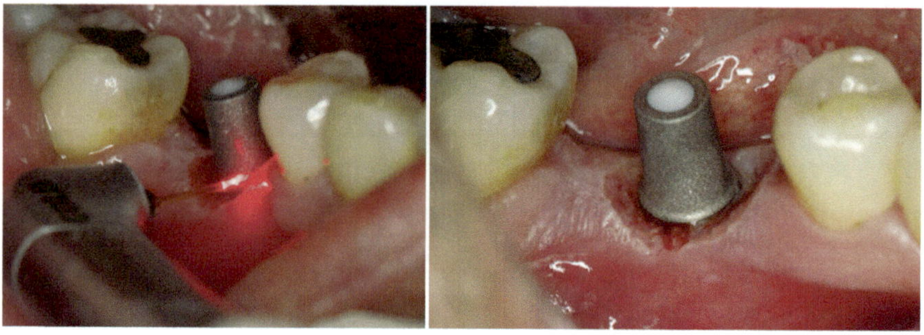

Fig. 7.39 Dental laser (Er,Cr:YSGG, Biolase) used to perform the second-stage procedure together with refining peri-implant soft tissue contour

7.4.5 Impression Coping

After creating an acceptable emergence profile and soft tissue contour by using a custom-made healing abutment or temporary crown, the soft tissue contour should be copied to the cast sent to the technician to design the final restoration with a similar emergence profile to that of the shaped and contoured soft tissue. Impression copings (transfer copings) can be customized intraorally by adding flowable composite to match the shape of the peri-implant soft tissue [39, 40]. An alternative technique would be to make the impression while the contoured provisional restoration is in place on the implant. The restoration is later unscrewed, and an analog is attached to it and reinserted into the impression that is poured. After unscrewing the provisional restoration, an accurate imprint of the contoured soft tissue is duplicated on the cast [41]. This would help the dental technician to fabricate a restoration with a similar emergence profile to the one that had already been made (Fig. 7.40a–e).

7.4.6 Abutment Selection

Stock abutments, whether screw or cement retained, are usually supplied with a round cross-section of different diameters and collar heights. An abutment of appropriate diameter should be selected to match the diameter of the tooth to be restored. This way, a proper emergence profile can be created (Fig. 7.41) [42]. Custom-made abutments can be constructed by using different materials, most commonly tooth-colored ones to avoid metal display, especially in cases with a thin peri-implant soft tissue biotype [43]. Custom-made abutments can be constructed by using conventional techniques or CAD-CAM technology. They offer many advantages over stock ones. Most important is the ability to create a custom emergence profile that guides

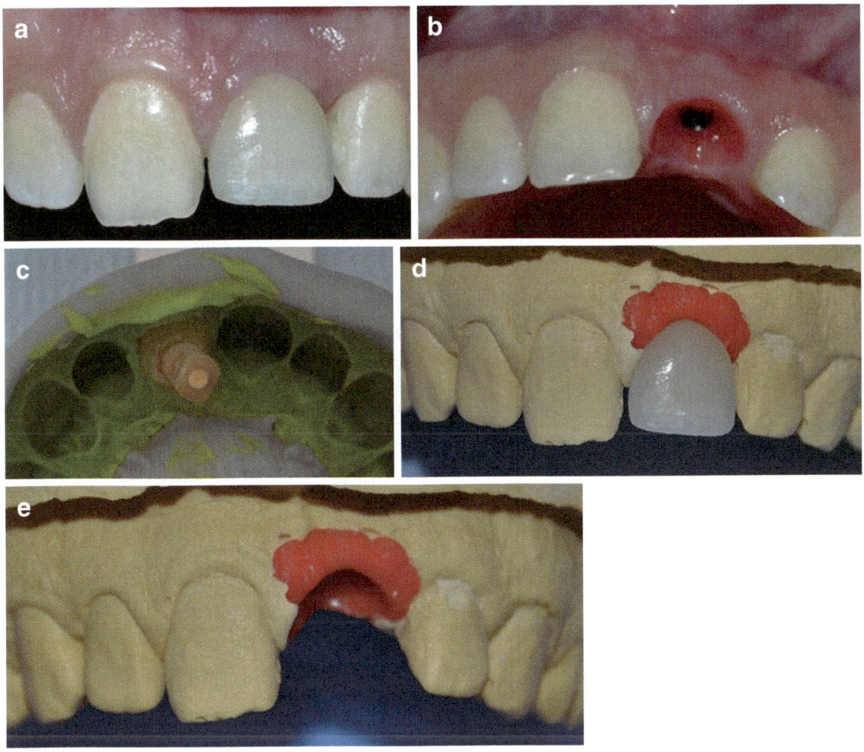

Fig. 7.40 (**a**) Provisional restoration after final contouring, (**b**) Peri-implant soft tissue contoured by the provisional restoration, (**c**) Impression with the provisional restoration that is unscrewed from the patient mouth, implant analog attached to it and reinserted back into the impression. (**d**) Impression is poured. Gingival mask material is added, (**e**) Peri-implant soft tissue profile duplicated on the case

the gingival margin to a proper contour and the ability to create a custom finish line following the contour of the peri-implant soft tissue margin to be able to efficiently remove excess cement (Fig. 7.42a,b).

7.4.7 Final Restoration

A well-designed final restoration with a properly contoured emergence profile is essential to support peri-implant soft tissues, thus creating an esthetic gingival margin. Ultimate esthetic results with implants can be achieved by using tooth-colored, metal-free restorations (Fig. 7.43a–d).

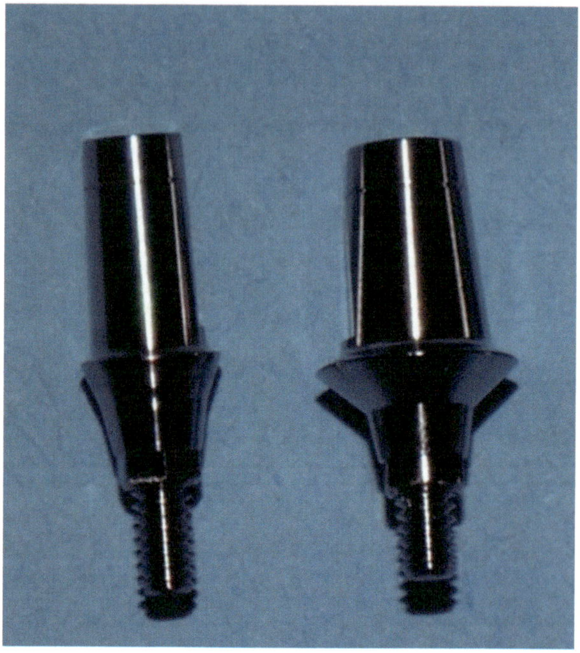

Fig. 7.41 Stock abutments are provided with different diameters selected according to the clinical situation

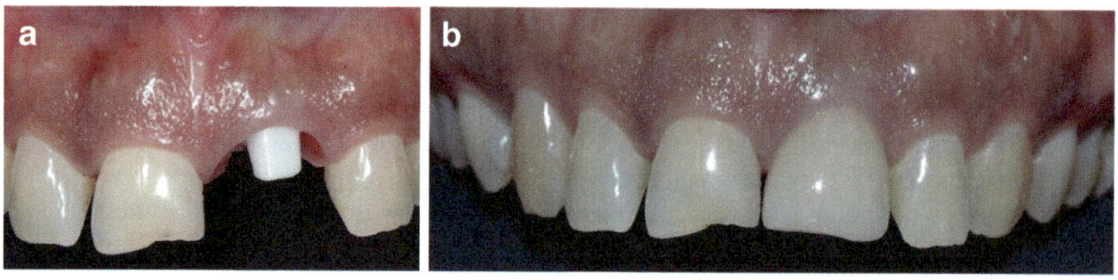

Fig. 7.42 (**a**) Tooth-colored zirconia abutment. (**b**) Lithium disilicate restoration with appropriate color match

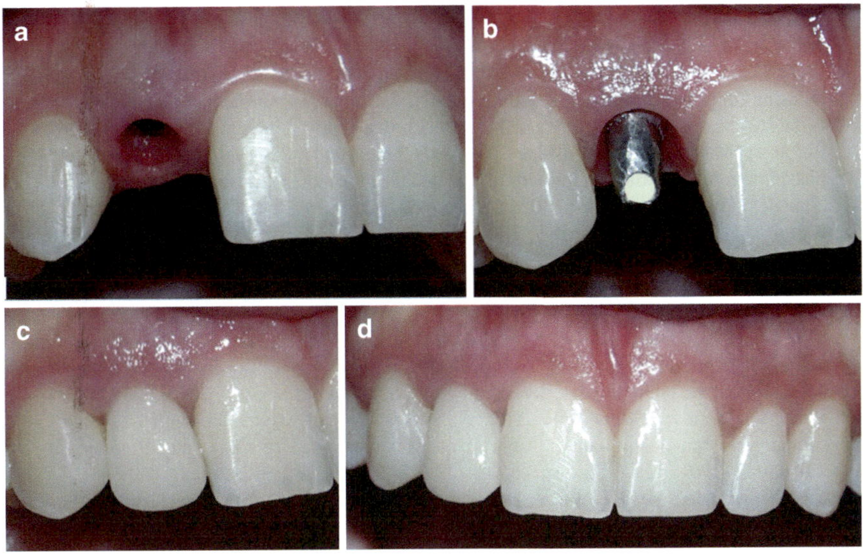

Fig. 7.43 (**a**) Properly positioned implant, (**b**) properly contoured peri-implant soft tissue margin by using a contoured conventional restoration, (**c**) all ceramic (lithium disilicate) final restoration with a suitable emergence profile, and (**d**) all ceramic (lithium disilicate) final restoration with a suitable emergence profile

References

1. Johnson K. A study of the dimensional changes occurring in the maxilla after tooth extraction. Part I. Normal healing. Aust Dent J. 1963;8:428–33.
2. Schropp L, et al. Bone healing and soft tissue contour changes following single-tooth extraction: a clinical and radiographic 12-month prospective study. Int J Periodontics Restorative Dent. 2003;23(4):313–23.
3. Johnson K. A study of the dimensional changes occurring in the maxilla following tooth extraction. Aust Dent J. 1969;14:241–4.
4. Cattoni F, Chirico L, Merlone A, Manacorda M, Vinci R, Gherlone EF. Digital smile designed computer-aided surgery versus traditional workflow in "all on four" rehabilitations: a randomized clinical trial with 4-years follow-up. Int J Environ Res Public Health. 2021;18(7):3449. https://doi.org/10.3390/ijerph18073449. PMID: 33810379; PMCID: PMC8037328.
5. Ramadan RE, Bahgat MM, Abdelhamid AM, Khamis MM. Registration of maxillomandibular relationship through a fully digital workflow for complete-mouth rehabilitation with screw-retained fixed implant-supported prostheses: a clinical report. J Prosthet Dent. 2023;S0022-3913(22):00760. https://doi.org/10.1016/j.prosdent.2022.11.027.
6. Gadallah MA, Aboelsayed KM, Neena AF, Khamis MM. Digitally empowered esthetic dentistry "functionally and biologically driven digital smile design". Alex Dent J. 2023;47:24. https://doi.org/10.21608/adjalexu.2023.273772.

7. D'Souza KM, Aras MA. Types of implant surgical guides in dentistry: a review. J Oral Implantol. 2012;38:643–52.
8. Sarhan MM, Khamis MM, El-Sharkawy AM. Evaluation of the accuracy of implant placement by using fully guided versus partially guided tissue supported surgical guides with cylindrical versus C-shaped guiding holes: a split-mouth clinical study. J Prosthet Dent. 2021;125:620–7.
9. Elkomy MM, Khamis MM, El-Sharkawy AM. Clinical and radiographic evaluation of implants placed with fully guided versus partially guided tissue-supported surgical guides: a split mouth clinical study. J Prosthet Dent. 2021;126:58–66.
10. Kammoun YA, Khamis MM, El-Sharkawy AM, Fahmy RA. Radiographic assessment of bone level changes around four implants supporting immediately loaded mandibular screw-retained prosthesis. Alex Dent J. 2022;47:113. https://doi.org/10.21608/ADJALEXU.2021.47381.1114.
11. Mohamed LA, Khamis MM, El-Sharkawy AM, Fahmy RA. Evaluation of immediately loaded mandibular four vertical versus tilted posterior implants supporting fixed detachable restorations without versus with posterior cantilevers. Oral Maxillofac Surg. 2022;26:373–81.
12. Buser D, Mericske-Stern R, Dula K, Lang NP. Clinical experience with one-stage, non-submerged dental implants. Adv Dent Res. 1999;13:153–61. https://doi.org/10.1177/08959374990130010501.
13. Macedo JP, Pereira J, Vahey BR, Henriques B, Benfatti CAM, Magini RS, López-López J, Souza JCM. Morse taper dental implants and platform switching: the new paradigm in oral implantology. Eur J Dent. 2016;10(1):148–54. https://doi.org/10.4103/1305-7456.175677. PMID: 27011755; PMCID: PMC4784146.
14. Todescan FF, et al. Influence of the microgap in the peri-implant hard and soft tissues: a histomorphometric study in dogs. Int J Oral Maxillofac Implants. 2002;17:467–72.
15. Liu Y, Wang J. Influences of microgap and micromotion of implant-abutment interface on marginal bone loss around implant neck. Arch Oral Biol. 2017;83:153–60.
16. King GN, Hermann JS, Schoolfield JD, Buser D, Cochran DL. Influence of the size of the microgap on crestal bone levels in non-submerged dental implants: a radiographic study in the canine mandible. J Periodontol. 2002;73:1111–7.
17. Roehling S, Schlegel KA, Woelfler H, Gahlert M. Zirconia compared to titanium dental implants in preclinical studies-a systematic review and meta-analysis. Clin Oral Implants Res. 2019;30(5):365–95. https://doi.org/10.1111/clr.13425. Epub 2019 Apr 16.
18. Chu SJ, Kan JY, Lee EA, Lin GH, Jahangiri L, Nevins M, Wang HL. Restorative emergence profile for single-tooth implants in healthy periodontal patients: clinical guidelines and decision-making strategies. Int J Periodontics Restorative Dent. 2019;40:19–29. https://doi.org/10.11607/prd.3697.
19. El-Danasory MB, Khamis MM, Hakim AAA, Fahmy RA. CAD-CAM custom healing abutments: a dental technique. J Prosthet Dent. 2022;S0022–3913:00638. https://doi.org/10.1016/j.prosdent.2022.09.019.
20. Engelman MJ. Clinical decision making and treatment planning in osseointegration. Batavia, IL: Quintessence Publishing; 1996.
21. Al-Harbi SA. Nonsurgical management of interdental papilla associated with multiple maxillary anterior implants: a clinical report. J Prosthet Dent. 2005;93:212–6.
22. Tarnow DP, Magner AW, Fletcher P. The effect of the distance from the contact point to the crest of bone on the presence or absence of the interproximal dental papilla. J Periodontol. 1992;63(12):995–6. https://doi.org/10.1902/jop.1992.63.12.995.
23. Sailer I, Karasan D, Todorovic A, Ligoutsikou M, Pjetursson BE. Prosthetic failures in dental implant therapy. Periodontol 2000. 2022;88(1):130–44. https://doi.org/10.1111/prd.12416. PMID: 35103329; PMCID: PMC9305548.
24. Ramanauskaite A, Sader R. Esthetic complications in implant dentistry. Periodontol 2000. 2022;88(1):73–85. https://doi.org/10.1111/prd.12412.
25. Esquivel J, Meda RG, Blatz MB. The impact of 3D implant position on emergence profile design. Int J Periodontics Restorative Dent. 2021;41(1):79–86. https://doi.org/10.11607/prd.5126.

26. Bhola M, Neely AL, Kolhatkar S. Immediate implant placement: clinical decisions, advantages, and disadvantages. J Prosthodont. 2008;17(7):576–81. https://doi.org/10.1111/j.1532-849X.2008.00359.x. Epub 2008 Aug 26.
27. Chu SJ, Salama MA, Salama H, Garber DA, Saito H, Sarnachiaro GO, Tarnow DP. The dual-zone therapeutic concept of managing immediate implant placement and provisional restoration in anterior extraction sockets. Compend Contin Educ Dent. 2012;33(524–532):534.
28. Ruales-Carrera E, Pauletto P, Apaza-Bedoya K, Volpato CA, Özcan M, Benfatti CA. Peri-implant tissue management after immediate implant placement using a customized healing abutment. J Esthet Restor Dent. 2019;31:533e541.
29. Akin R. A new concept in maintaining the emergence profile in immediate posterior implant placement: the anatomic harmony abutment. J Oral Maxillofac Surg. 2016;74:2385e2392.
30. Campaner M, Takamiya AS, Bitencourt SB, et al. Cytotoxicity and inflammatory response of different types of provisional restorative materials. Arch Oral Biol. 2020;111:104643.
31. Linkevicius T, Puisys A, Linkevicius R, Alkimaviciu J, Ginevici E, Limnhevicicene L. The influence of submerged healing abutment or subcrestal implant placement on soft tissue thickness and crestal bone stability. A 2-year randomized clinical trial. Clin Implant Dent Relat Res. 2020;22:497–506.
32. Schuler DE. Use of the laser in the oral cavity. Otolaryngol Clin N Am. 1990;23:31–42.
33. Khamis MM, Abdelrehim AA. Interdisciplinary management of a patient with a gummy smile. J Oral Maxillofac Radiol. 2019;7:38–43.
34. Rizoiu, et al. Effects of an erbium, chromium: yttrium, scandium, gallium, garnet laser on mucocutaneous soft tissues. Oral Surg Oral Med Oral Pathol Oral Radiol Endod. 1996;82:386–95.
35. Tunc SK, Yayli NZ, Talmac AC, Feslihan E, Akbal D. Clinical comparison of the use of ER,CR:YSGG and diode lasers in second stage implants surgery. Saudi Med J. 2019;40(5):490–8. https://doi.org/10.15537/smj.2019.5.24105. PMID: 31056627; PMCID: PMC6535160.
36. Ramadan RE, Segan L, Abdelhamid AM, Khamis MM. Gingival melanin depigmentation with 4 different laser wavelengths 445, 940, 1064 and 2940nm: a case report. Alex Dent J. 2022;47:27. https://doi.org/10.21608/adjalexu.2023.273862.
37. Ashry A, Khamis MM, Abdelhamid AM, Segaan LG. Lip repositioning and guided gingivectomy combined treatment for excessive gingival display by using 940-nm diode laser: a case report. Laser Dent Sci. 2023;7:25. https://doi.org/10.1007/s41547-023-00174-5.
38. Troedhan A, Mahmoud ZT, Wainwright M, Khamis MM. Cutting bone with drills, burs, lasers and piezotomes: a comprehensive systematic review and recommendations for the clinician. Int J Oral Craniofac Sci. 2017;3(2):020–33. https://doi.org/10.17352/2455-4634.0000128.
39. Buskin R, Salinas TJ. Transferring emergence profile created from the provisional to the definitive restoration. Pract Periodontics Aesthet Dent. 1998;10:1171–9.
40. Stumpel J, Haechler W, Bedrossian E. Customized abutments to shape and transfer peri-implant soft-tissue contours. J Calif Dent Assoc. 2000;28:301–9.
41. Tsai BY. A method for obtaining peri-implant soft-tissue contours by using screw-retained provisional restorations as impression copings: a clinical report. J Oral Implantol. 2011;37(5):605–9.
42. Khamis MM, Zakaria NH. Effect of screw access channel on fracture resistance of lithium disilicate cement retained implant supported posterior crowns. J Prosthet Dent. 2022;127:618–25.
43. Farrag KM, Khamis MM. Effect of anodized abutment collars on peri-implant soft tissue: a split-mouth clinical study. J Prosthet Dent. 2021;130(1):59–67.

8 Prosthetic Role in Peri-implant Soft Tissue Management: Prosthetic Phase

Mohamed Moataz Khamis

8.1 Restoration Design (Screw Vs. Cement Retention)

Fixed implant restorations can either be screw or cement retained (Fig. 8.1). Each design has its merits and drawbacks. Screw-retained restorations are retrievable. Retightening a loose abutment screw can therefore be performed easily. They do not depend on cement for retention. Therefore, the problem of removing excess cement

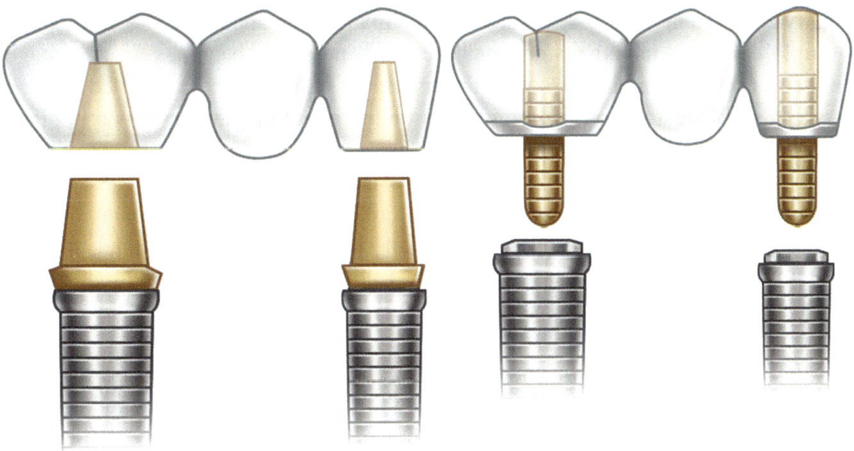

Fig. 8.1 Fixed implant restorations can either be screw or cement retained

M. M. Khamis (✉)
Department of Prosthodontics, Faculty of Dentistry, Alexandria University, Alexandria, Egypt

M. Hassan (ed.), *Peri-Implant Soft Tissue Management*,
https://doi.org/10.1007/978-3-031-45516-2_8

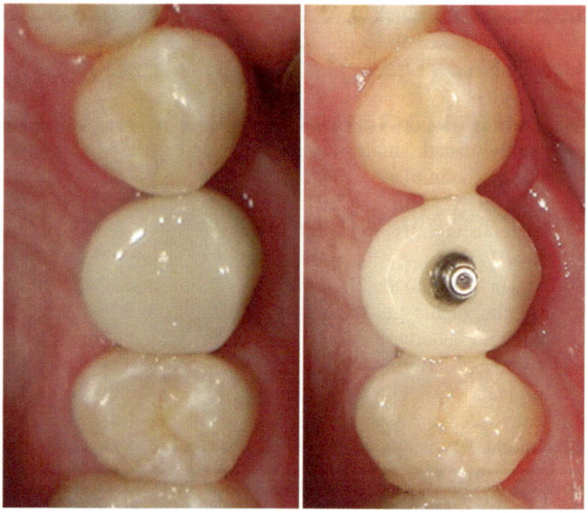

Fig. 8.2 Screw access channels can interfere with occlusal contacts

does not exist. However, they require special technical skills and are usually more expensive than cement-retained restorations as they may require additional components and procedures [1].

Cement-retained restorations do not have a screw access channel; therefore, they are more esthetic and provide better occlusal anatomy contacts (Fig. 8.2). They are usually easier to fabricate especially if ready-made stock abutments are used. When multiple cement-retained restorations are used, passivity becomes an advantage. The presence of a cement gap space, the amount of which can be controlled, ensures passivity of the restoration, which is important to avoid undue stresses on implants when abutment screws are tightened [1]. However, if excess cement is not completely removed, adverse peri-implant soft tissue reactions can occur [2].

The choice between screw and cement retention depends on many factors, including interocclusal distance, location of the screw access channel, esthetic demands, need for restoration retrievability, frequency of screw loosening, laboratory efficiency, need for passivity of fit, combining natural tooth and implant support, and finish line location [3–6].

It is important to mention that the choice between using a screw- or cement-retained restoration should be decided during the treatment plan phase and not after implant placement. Most of the factors of choice between both designs can be determined during treatment planning. Therefore, the restoration design and means of retention are always predetermined, and the treatment plan and implant positioning and alignment are always geared toward achieving a predictable restoration.

8.1.1 Interocclusal Distance

The bond strength of cement retention depends on several factors, the most important being the surface area for cement bonding [7, 8]. The larger the surface of the abutment, the greater the bond strength between the abutment and restoration.

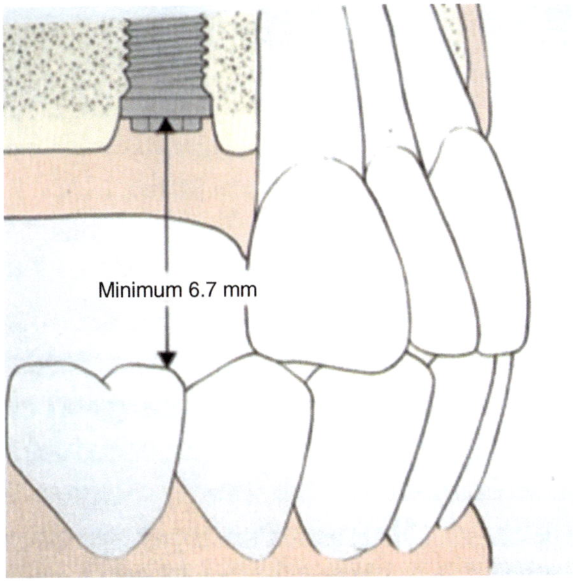

Fig. 8.3 Manufacturers recommend a minimum inter-arch distance for screw-retained abutments that should be checked during treatment planning

Generally, in cases with a wide inter-arch distance allowing for a longer abutment, screw and cement retention are equally acceptable. However, in cases with narrow inter-arch distance, screw retention is more favorable as it depends on the tightness of the abutment/restoration screw rather than abutment surface area [3, 9].

Unlike cement-retained abutments, those for screw retention usually cannot be modified or shortened. Interarch distance should therefore be measured, and the minimal height of a screw-retained abutment should be selected according to manufacturer guidelines (Fig. 8.3).

8.1.2 Location of the Screw Access Channel

Screw-retained restorations require a screw access channel that should be located on the palatal surface of anterior teeth (Fig. 8.4) and in the center of the occlusal surface of posterior teeth (Fig. 8.5) so as not to interfere with the esthetic and biomechanical qualities of the restoration. Screw access channels are usually blocked with the composite resin of a similar shade to the restoration (Fig. 8.6).

However, the shade of the composite does not always match the shade of the restoration, especially if the restoration has a metal component, such as porcelain fused to metal. The shadow of the metal usually interferes with the esthetic qualities of the restoration (Fig. 8.7). Locating a screw access channel on an incisal edge or a functional cusp tip might weaken the restoration and therefore should be avoided (Fig. 8.8). This requires implants to be properly aligned during placement to ensure a favorable access hole location. An alternative would be to use angled screw-retained abutments or cement-retained restorations that do not have a screw access channel on the final restoration.

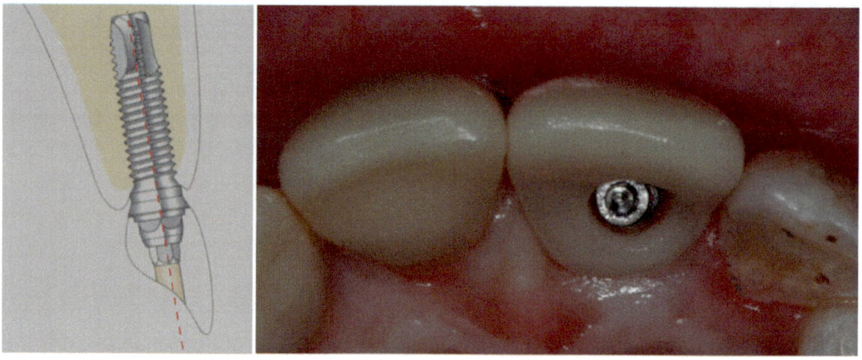

Fig. 8.4 Screw access channel ideally located on the palatal surface of anterior teeth

Fig. 8.5 Screw access channel ideally located in the center of the occlusal surface of posterior teeth

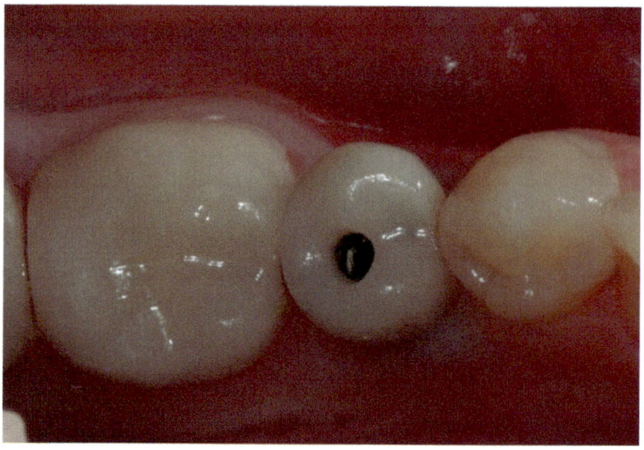

Fig. 8.6 Screw access channel blocked with composite resin

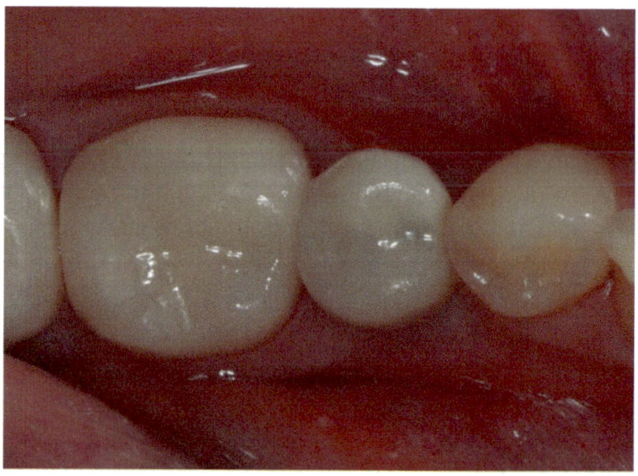

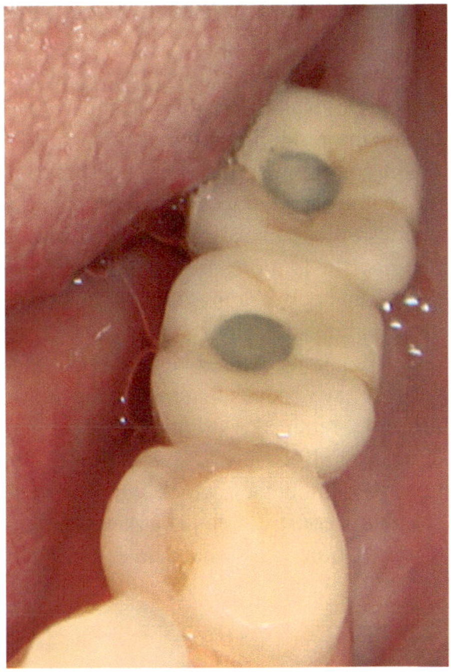

Fig. 8.7 The shadow of the metal appearing through the composite interfering with the esthetic qualities of the restoration

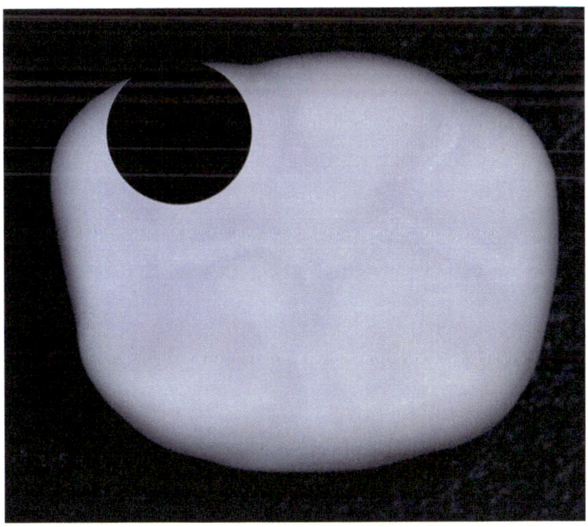

Fig. 8.8 Screw access channel should not be located on an incisal edge or a functional cusp so as not to weaken the restoration

8.1.3 Abutment/Restoration Finish Line Position

Abutment/restoration finish line location can either be supragingival, subgingival, or equigingival. Supragingival finish lines have many advantages. They are easier during impression making as there would be no need for soft tissue retraction that might compromise peri-implant soft tissue attachment [10, 11]. Peri-implant soft tissue does not collapse between visits if a temporary restoration is not used, finish line visibility makes lab work procedures simpler, detection of restoration abutment marginal fit is more predictable, and excess cement can easily be removed. The main drawback of supragingival finish lines is the unesthetic appearance of the abutment collar especially if a metal abutment is used (Fig. 8.9).

For cement-retained restorations, excess cement can be completely removed without any residues that may compromise the peri-implant soft tissue health. Even for screw-retained restorations, supragingival finish lines are preferable from a biological point of view. A micro gap always exists at the abutment restoration junction, the amount of which varies depending on the technique and accuracy of prosthesis construction [12]. A micro gap of considerable size that may result from a restoration with inaccurate margins can harbor bacteria that may cause

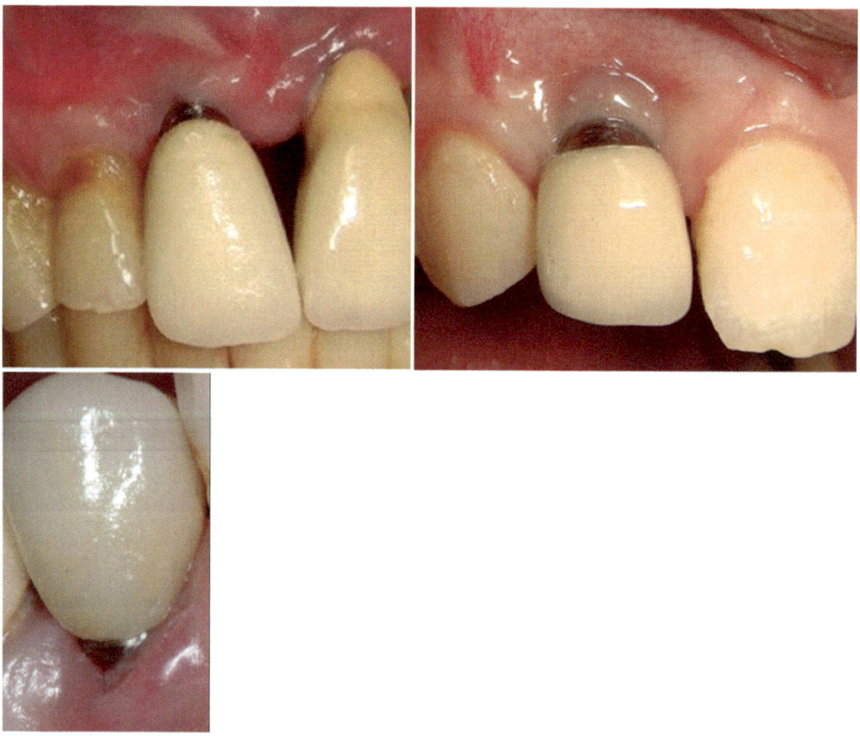

Fig. 8.9 Supragingival finish lines are inappropriate in the esthetic zone, especially with metal abutments

peri-implant soft tissue problems. Supragingival location of the micro gap is therefore desirable. When selecting a supragingival finish line, both designs would be similar from a biological point of view.

To reduce the amount of micro gap between prosthetic components, it is always recommended to torque the abutment screw according to manufacturer's instructions by using a torque wrench. According to studies, this significantly reduces the micro gap and consequently peri-implant soft tissue problems [13].

Subgingival finish lines are mainly indicated in the esthetic zone to avoid abutment collar display that can compromise esthetics, especially if a metal abutment is used. In such cases, the subgingival depth of the finish line must be controlled to avoid peri-implant soft and hard tissue problems.

8.1.3.1 Cement-Retained Restorations with a Screw Access Channel

Cement-retained restorations have many advantages; however, the difficulty encountered in the complete removal of excess cement precludes their routine use. To solve the problem of excess cement, a modified cement-retained restoration was advocated combining the advantages of screw and cement retention [14]. The modification involves the creation of a screw access channel on the occlusal surface of the cement-retained restoration (Fig. 8.10). After complete intraoral cementation (Fig. 8.11), the restoration/abutment assembly can be removed by unscrewing the abutment screw through the screw access channel and the excess cement can be completely removed extra orally (Fig. 8.12a–c). The restoration after cementation becomes permanently attached to the abutment and can be screw retained onto the implant. The screw access channel can later on be filled with a composite of similar shade [1] (Fig. 8.13a,b).

The advantage of this design is that it combines the benefits of both screw and cement retention. The limitations, however, include that it is not recommended if

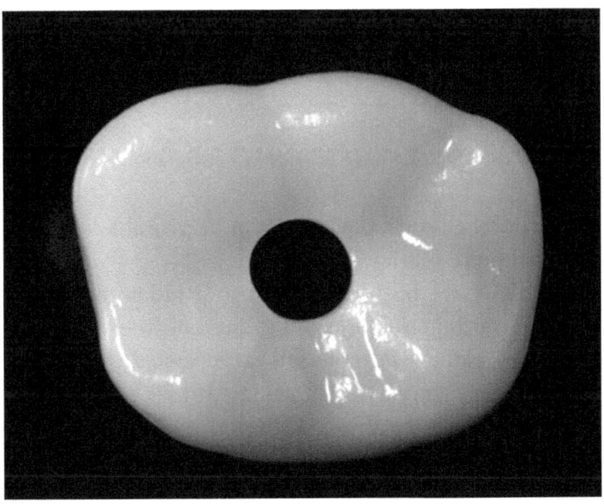

Fig. 8.10 Screw access channel on the occlusal surface of the restoration

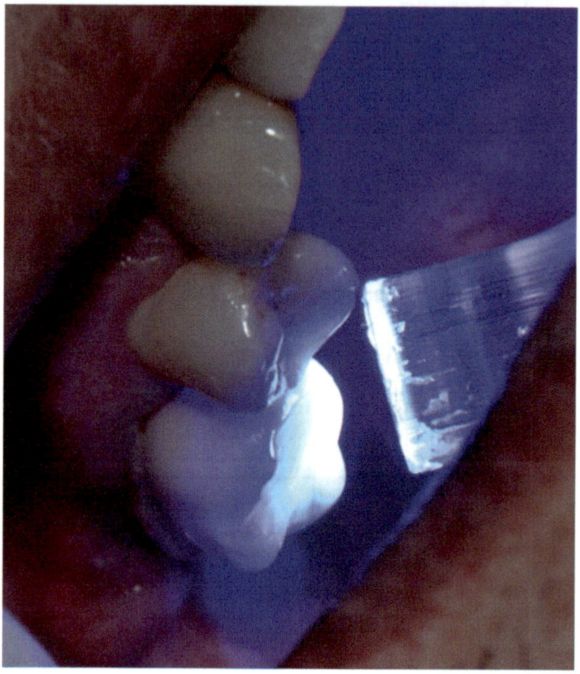

Fig. 8.11 Restoration cemented on abutment by using light cure resin cement

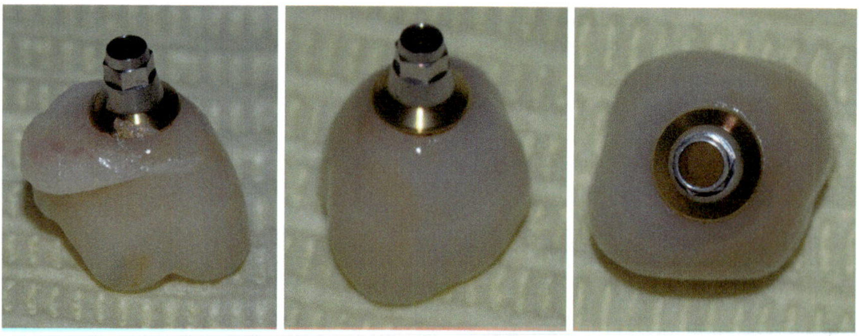

Fig. 8.12 Restoration unscrewed after cementation and excess cement completely removed

the screw access channel is not in a favorable position from an esthetic or biomechanical point of view (Fig. 8.14).

Studies have been conducted to evaluate the effect of creating a screw access channel on the structural durability and the fracture resistance of the restoration. Different restorative materials were tested, including zirconia, lithium disilicate, and porcelain fused to metal [1, 15–17]. In spite of the variability of the results between various studies and tested materials, most of the studies did not show

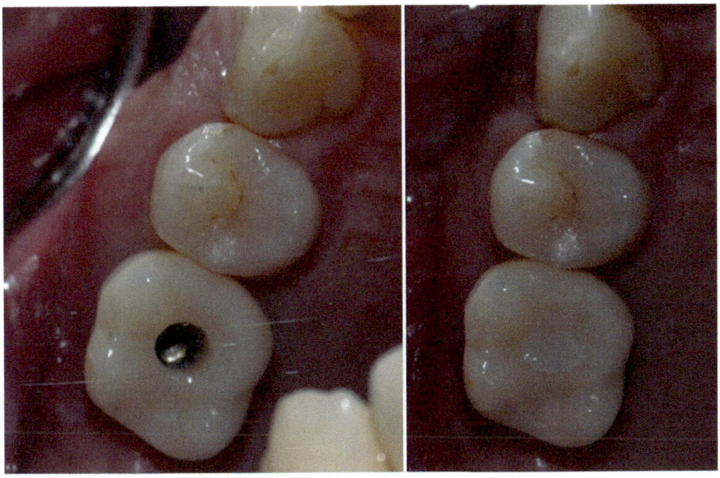

Fig. 8.13 Screw access channel closed with composite resin of appropriate shade

Fig. 8.14 Screw access channel should not be created on the labial or buccal surface of teeth, especially in the esthetic zone

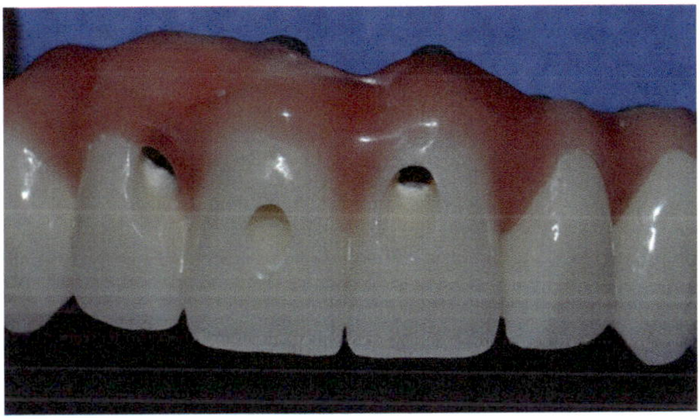

significant weakening of the restorations. In multiunit restorations where passivity of the restoration is of utmost importance, this technique can also be applied provided that implants are parallel or very close to being parallel [18–20] (Fig. 8.15a,b).

8.1.3.2 Peri-implant Soft Tissue Thickness/Finish Line Location

Locating the finish line in the desired position is achieved by first measuring the peri-implant soft tissue thickness from the implant platform to the free gingival margin, then selecting an abutment with a suitable collar height that can be shorter than the soft tissue thickness to position the finish line subgingivally or greater than the soft tissue thickness to position the finish line supragingivally. It is therefore important to give the soft tissue a chance to heal and stabilize after second-stage surgery to be able to properly locate the restoration finish line [21] (Fig. 8.16). Measuring peri-implant soft tissue thickness can be performed by using many instruments, the easiest of which is a plastic periodontal probe (Fig. 8.17).

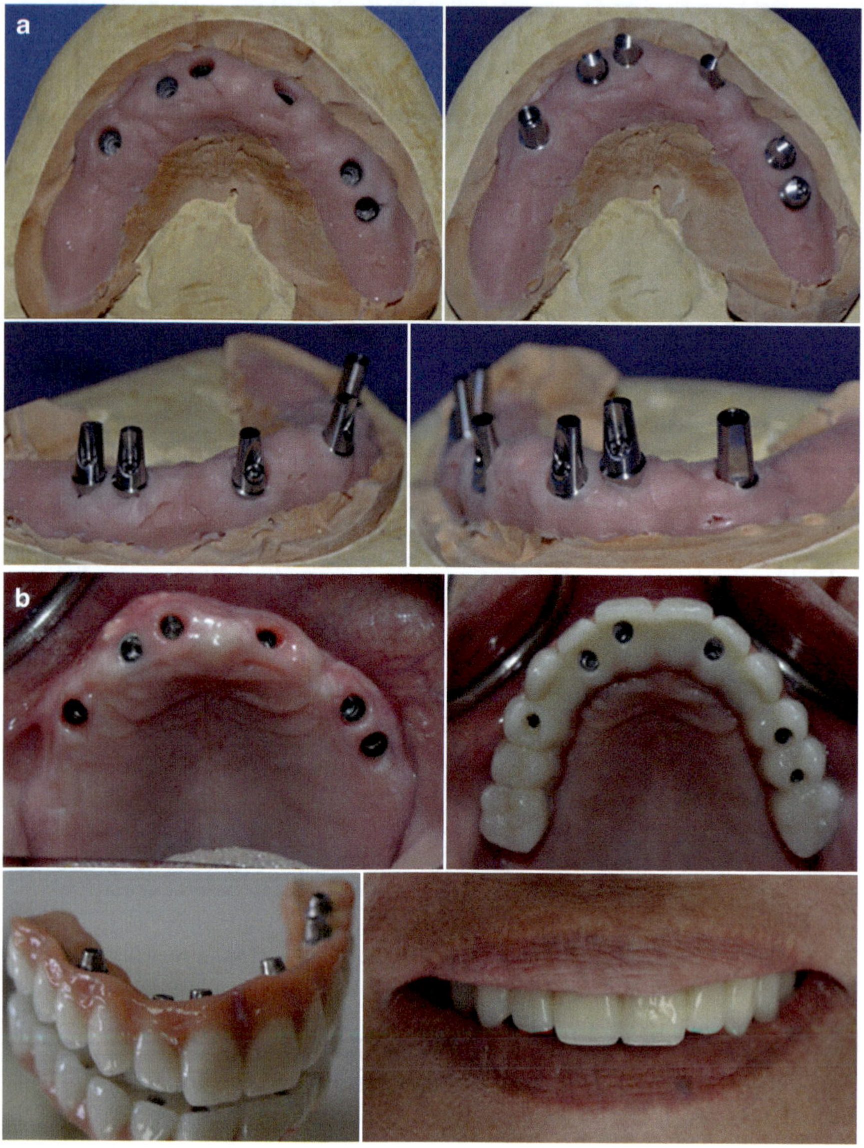

Fig. 8.15 (**a**) Cement retention provides passivity with multiunit restorations, especially when abutments are parallel. (**b**) Screw access channels in favorable positions not interfering with the esthetic or biomechanical properties of the restoration

Cement-retained restorations have always been guilty of causing peri-implant soft tissue irritation and inflammation due to the excess cement that is difficult to completely remove. The main cause of peri-implant soft tissue problems associated with cement-retained restorations is the inappropriate finish line location resulting

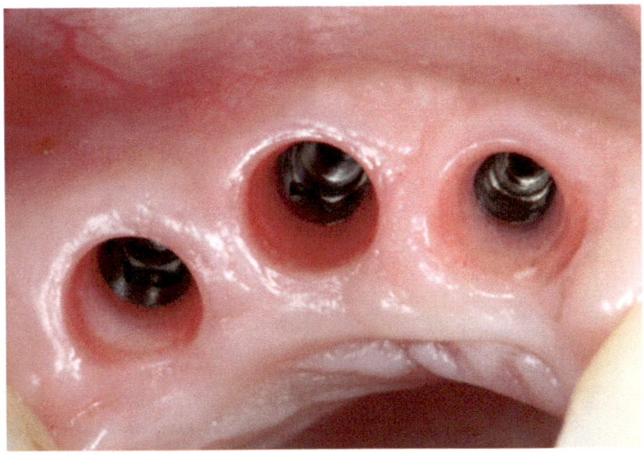

Fig. 8.16 Soft tissue healing following second-stage surgery

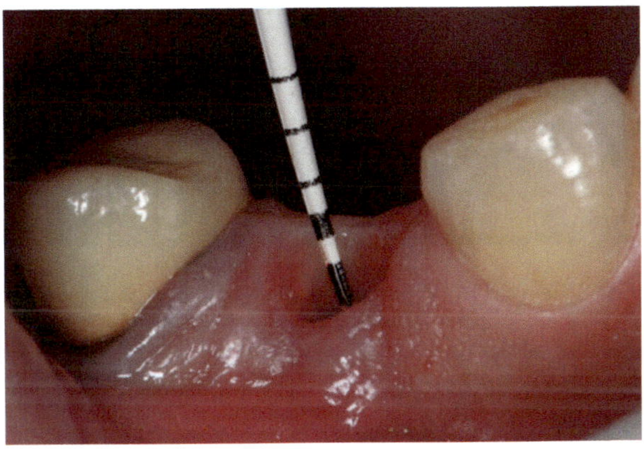

Fig. 8.17 Measuring peri-implant soft tissue thickness by using a plastic periodontal probe

from improper abutment collar height selection or designing. A cement-retained restoration with a supragingival finish line does not cause any soft tissue problems as excess cement can be completely removed. Even if a 1 mm subgingival finish line is used, excess cement can still be removed conveniently. However, in the case of deep subgingival finish lines greater than 2 mm, excess cement removal becomes very difficult, especially interproximally, as it is associated with bleeding and pain preventing proper cement removal. Residual cement causes peri-implant soft tissue problems that can advance to peri-implantitis [2] (Fig. 8.18).

8.1.3.3 Relation Between Finish Line Contour and Peri-implant Soft Tissue Contour

Measuring peri-implant soft tissue thickness is usually performed at the midfacial region. However, peri-implant soft tissue thickness may vary between the midfacial and interproximal regions. The difference would be less in cases associated with loss of interdental papillae and more in cases with well-preserved interdental papillae (Fig. 8.19a,b).

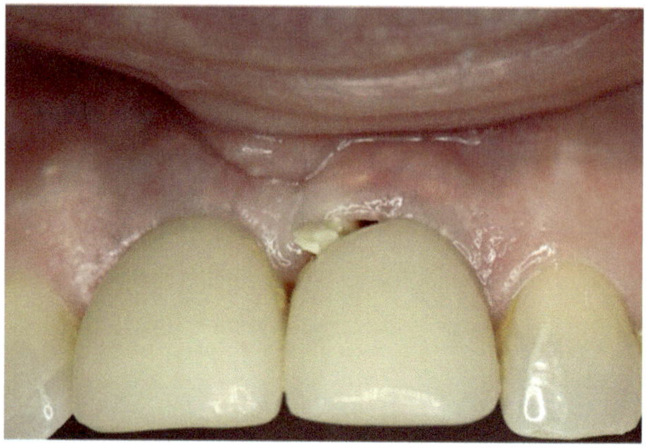

Fig. 8.18 Excess cement associated with a deep subgingival finish line

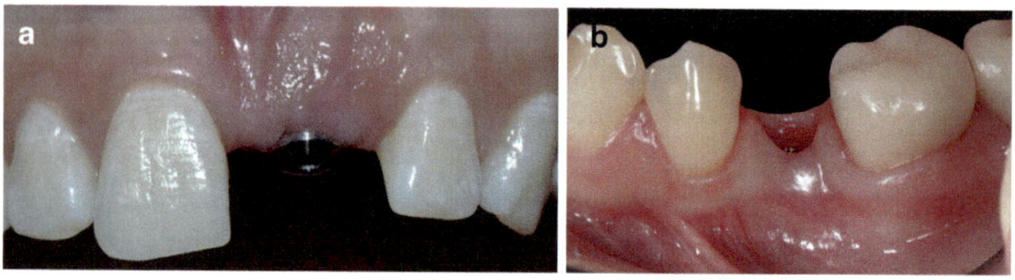

Fig. 8.19 (**a**) Flat peri-implant soft tissue margin associated with loss of interdental papillae. (**b**) Curved peri-implant soft tissue margin associated with well-preserved interdental papillae

Stock abutments usually have a finish line that has a straight contour. To achieve a 1-mm subgingival finish line position, the abutment collar height should be 1 mm shorter than the peri-implant mucosa thickness at the midfacial region. The problem usually exists at the proximal surfaces, where the 1-mm subgingival midfacial finish line becomes much deeper interproximally due to the thicker peri-implant mucosa at the interdental papilla region (Fig. 8.20a,b). When cement-retained restorations are used over stock abutments with a 1-mm subgingival midfacial finish line, excess cement would be easily removed facially but would be very difficult to remove interproximally. In such cases, custom-made cement-retained abutments are preferred and recommended [22, 23] (Fig. 8.21). Stock abutments can be acceptably used in cases with missing interdental papillae where the soft tissue contour is flat rather than curved (Fig. 8.16).

Custom-made abutments can be constructed by using conventional techniques or CAD-CAM technology. They can have a custom-made emergence profile together with a finish line contour that matches the peri-implant soft tissue contour. A 1-mm subgingival finish line can be maintained all around the restoration margins, making excess cement removal feasible and predictable (Fig. 8.21).

Screw-retained restorations are often preferred over cement-retained ones from a peri-implant soft tissue health point of view. Excess cement, when not completely removed, has always been a frequent reason for peri-implant soft and hard tissue

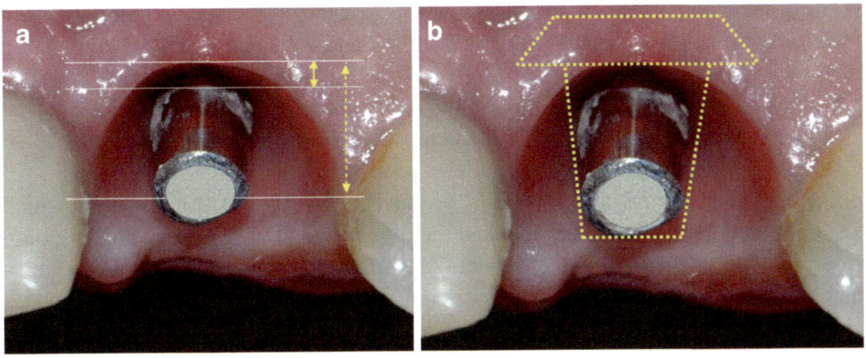

Fig. 8.20 (**a**) Peri-implant soft tissue thickness at the midfacial region is much less than at the interproximal region. (**b**) When using stock abutments with a flat finish line contour, excess cement would be very difficult to remove due to the thick interproximal soft tissue, making the finish line deep subgingivally

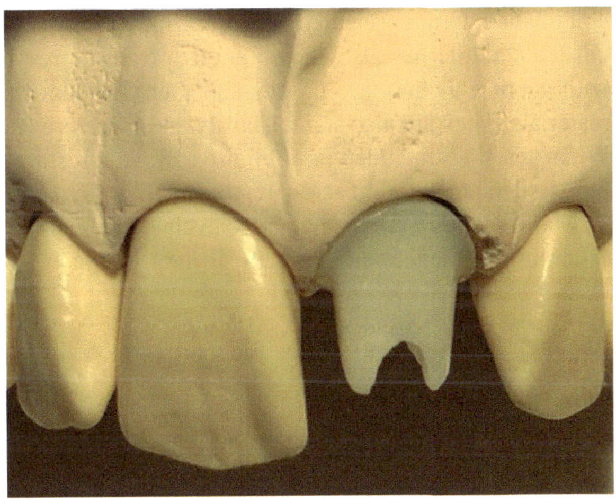

Fig. 8.21 Custom-made cement-retained abutments can have a finish line that follows the peri-implant soft tissue margin making excess cement removal more predictable

problems [2]. However, a big part of the problem is related to the location of the abutment restoration finish line. Properly constructed cement-retained restorations with proper finish line location can be as good as screw-retained ones.

8.2 Prosthetic Materials and Their Relation to Peri-implant Soft Tissue Health

The increasing demand for esthetic restorations has triggered the advancement and improvement of tooth-colored materials to match the high biomechanical and esthetic expectations. Tooth-colored materials are usually nonmetallic, either ceramic based or polymer based. However, metals are still being used with specific indications mainly related to their biomechanical superiority. Commonly used materials include metals such as gold, titanium, and cobalt chromium. Nonmetallic materials include ceramics, zirconia, resin nano ceramics, and BioHPP. Acrylics can also be used, however, mainly as temporary restorative materials [24, 25].

Implant restorations can be constructed by using conventional techniques or CAD-CAM technology that is taking over prosthodontics to a new dimension. All prosthetic materials are currently being produced for CAD-CAM fabrication, which has improved the accuracy and reduced the time needed for prosthesis construction. Improving the accuracy involves reducing the micro gap between prosthetic components that in turn improves the peri-implant soft tissue health and reduces complications.

The selection of prosthetic materials is usually based on many factors, including biomechanical, esthetic, and biological. Despite the importance of the biomechanical and esthetic features and properties of restorative materials, their biological interaction with peri-implant soft tissues is of major importance. In many situations, the prosthetic material becomes in direct contact with peri-implant soft tissues, especially with subgingival finish lines (Fig. 8.22).

Polished metals especially titanium have produced acceptable results [26, 27]. Glazed ceramic has also shown good soft tissue response [28]. Acrylics are used with caution as they are porous and therefore less hygienic than other definitive materials. They are also stained easily and therefore need to be changed frequently. When acrylic is included in a definitive implant restoration, it is always advisable to fabricate the restoration screw retained [3].

Many studies were conducted to evaluate the peri-implant soft tissue response to different prosthetic materials [29]. Brunot-Gohin et al. [30] investigated soft tissue

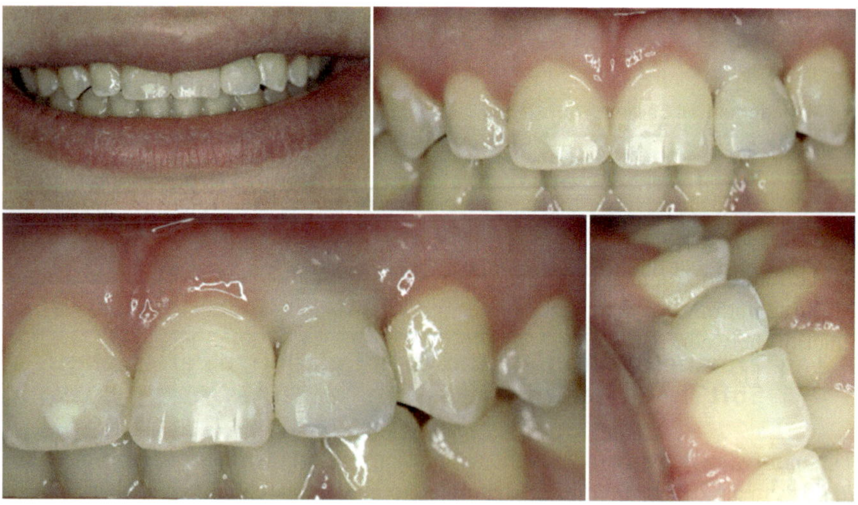

Fig. 8.22 With subgingival finish lines, restorative material becomes in direct contact with peri-implant soft tissues

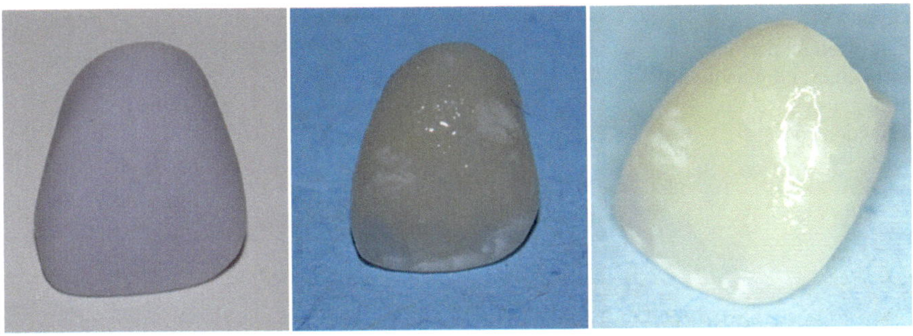

Fig. 8.23 Lithium disilicate restorative material. Can be polished or glazed

response to lithium disilicate with three different surface treatments: raw surface treatment, hand-polished surface treatment, and glazed surface treatment. Lithium disilicate polished ceramic provided better adhesion and proliferation than lithium disilicate glazed ceramic (Fig. 8.23). Van Brakel et al. [31] compared the peri-implant soft tissue response to titanium versus zirconia abutments. No differences in soft tissue health were seen in peri-implant mucosa adjacent to zirconia and titanium abutment surfaces. Similar results were demonstrated in an animal study by Blanco et al. [32], where peri-implant soft tissue response to implant abutments made of zirconia and titanium was similar after 9 months of healing.

8.2.1 CAD-CAM Technology

CAD-CAM technology has revolutionized prosthodontics. Digital workflows have replaced conventional procedures in almost all prosthetic work. The reason for that is that CAD-CAM technology improved the accuracy and predictability of prosthetic restorations and reduced the time and steps needed to fabricate restorations [23, 27, 33, 34]. The impact of CAD-CAM technology on peri-implant tissues is related to acquisition procedures together with marginal accuracy and passivity of restorations. Acquisition procedures involve digital impressions obtained by using scan bodies attached to implants or abutments [27, 34, 35]. When properly seated, scan bodies lightly retract peri-implant soft tissues, eliminating the need for soft tissue retraction associated with conventional impressions (Fig. 8.24).

Restorations performed by using CAD-CAM technology are machine dependent, eliminating the personal variation associated with dental technicians. Restoration margins and passivity are therefore more predictable with their positive impact on peri-implant soft and hard tissues [33, 36] (Fig. 8.25a,b).

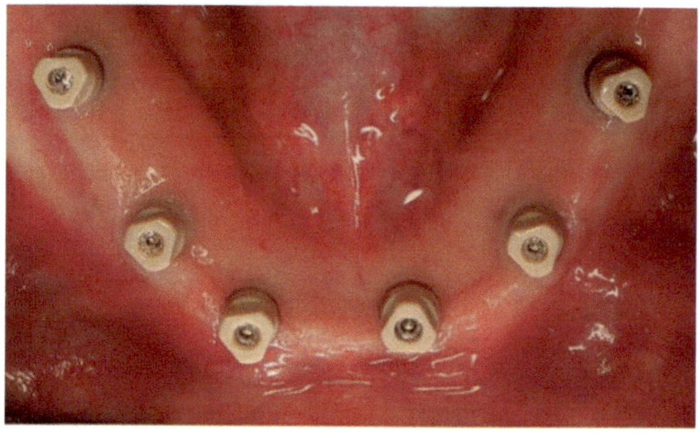

Fig. 8.24 Scan bodies lightly retract peri-implant soft tissues, eliminating the need to use a retraction cord

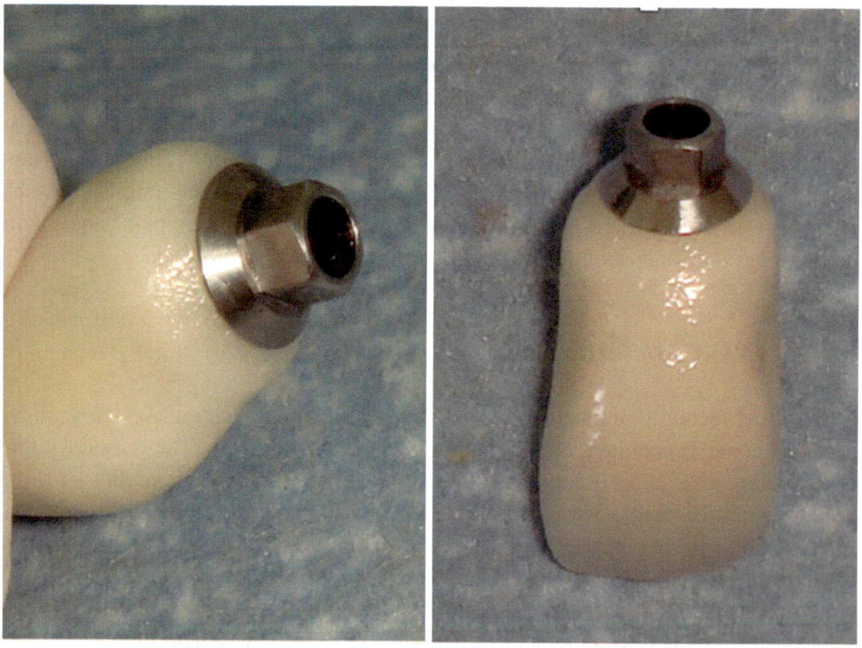

Fig. 8.25 CAD-CAM fabricated restorations have a precise marginal adaptation

8.2.2 Anodic Oxidation of Titanium Abutments

Titanium abutments have been used successfully over dental implants for many years. Peri-implant soft tissue response to polished titanium abutment collars has shown favorable results [37]. Their main drawback is their unesthetic color especially when used in the esthetic zone in cases with thin gingival biotype. Several attempts have been made to change the abutment color by using different materials and coatings. Gold, metal-ceramic, nitride-treated titanium, composite resin-coated titanium, thermal oxidation, chemical oxidation, and anodic-oxidized titanium have been used to mask the unesthetic grayish abutment color, especially the abutment collar [26, 38–43] (Fig. 8.26).

Anodic oxidation is a surface modification technique for changing the abutment color. Titanium is spontaneously coated with an oxide surface layer as soon as it is exposed to atmospheric air. Anodic oxidation promotes the production of a thick oxide surface layer based on the voltage used. Specific colors can be produced by controlling the variation in oxide layer thickness that interacts differently with light [44].

Studies have been conducted to evaluate the esthetic outcome of anodically oxidizing titanium abutment collars. Pink collars have been shown to improve gingival esthetics by masking the grayish titanium color [26, 43, 45] (Fig. 8.27a,b). In

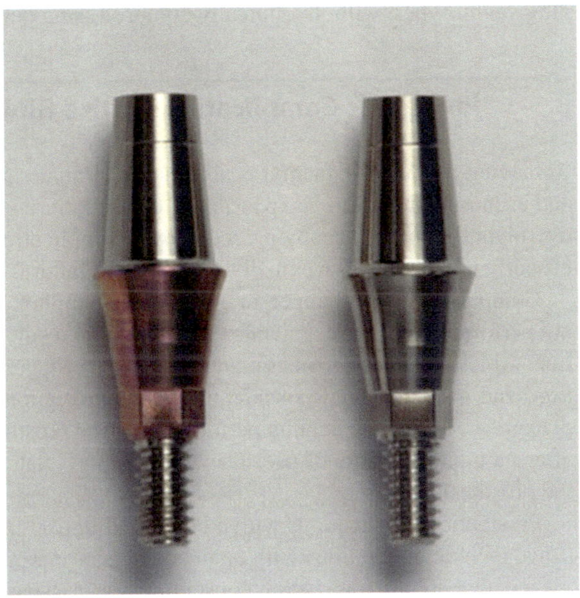

Fig. 8.26 Anodically oxidized abutment collar. The pink color masks the unesthetic grayish abutment color

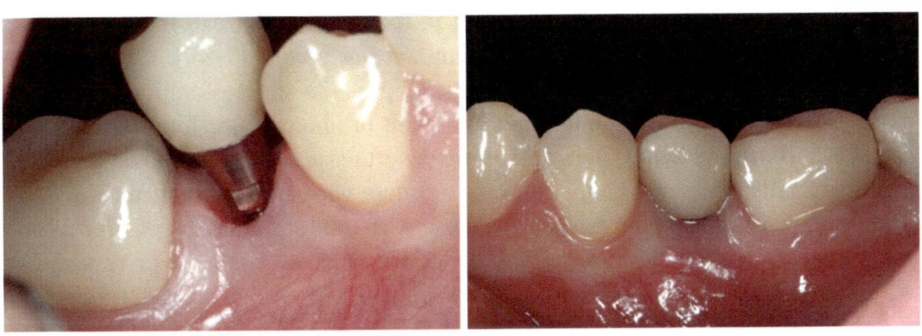

Fig. 8.27 Anodically oxidized pink abutment collar

addition, anodic oxidation alters the surface characteristics of titanium. Increasing the thickness of the surface oxide layer has also been reported to improve its surface hardness and corrosion resistance [46].

In an in vitro study, Wang et al. [45] reported that anodization increased the grain formation, surface roughness, and hydrophilicity of titanium. Although smooth machined titanium surfaces have been recommended for their improved soft tissue response, a degree of roughness is desirable. While the optimal degree of roughness is unclear, the proliferation of human gingival fibroblasts, their viability, and cell morphology have been reported to be similar on anodized and unanodized surfaces. In a split-mouth study, Farrag and Khamis [44] investigated the effect of anodized titanium on peri-implant soft tissue health and esthetics. Pink anodized titanium abutment collars did not produce a clinically significant effect on the health of peri-implant soft tissues. Anodic oxidation of titanium abutment collars is therefore an effective method to mask their grayish unesthetic color, especially in cases with thin gingival biotypes, without clinically compromising peri-implant soft tissues.

8.3 Prosthetic Complications with a Biological Impact

Achieving patient satisfaction is always the ultimate goal. However, complications and even implant failure are possible. Implant failure is not something that happens overnight. Failure is usually preceded by a complication that, if not recognized and properly handled, will eventually propagate to failure.

Complications can happen in every step of implant treatment if the procedure is not performed in a correct manner. Problems can result from improper patient selection, which involves prosthetic and surgical considerations, psychological evaluation, and even financial considerations. Complications can occur during implant placement, during the healing period, during the prosthetic procedures, and later on after months and years of use. They can also be related to the soft tissue, bone, or the prosthesis itself.

Prosthetic complications with a biological impact on peri-implant bone and soft tissue include restorations with open contacts or margins, improper occlusion, cantilevers that are too long, screw loosening, non-passive restorations, and connecting implants to natural teeth.

Restorations with open contacts result in food impaction, causing peri-implant soft tissue inflammation known as peri-implant mucositis [47–49]. If not properly treated, it can propagate to peri-implantitis (Fig. 8.28a–c). Restorations with open margins or micro gaps at the implant abutment or abutment restoration interfaces can also harbor food and bacteria, resulting in soft tissue problems and later on bone loss, especially if the restoration margins or micro gaps are subgingival (Fig. 8.29).

Restorations that are not passive, or those with too long cantilevers, or improper occlusion in the form of high points, deflective occlusal contacts, or restorations with sharp cusps can cause undue stress transmitted to the bone, causing bone

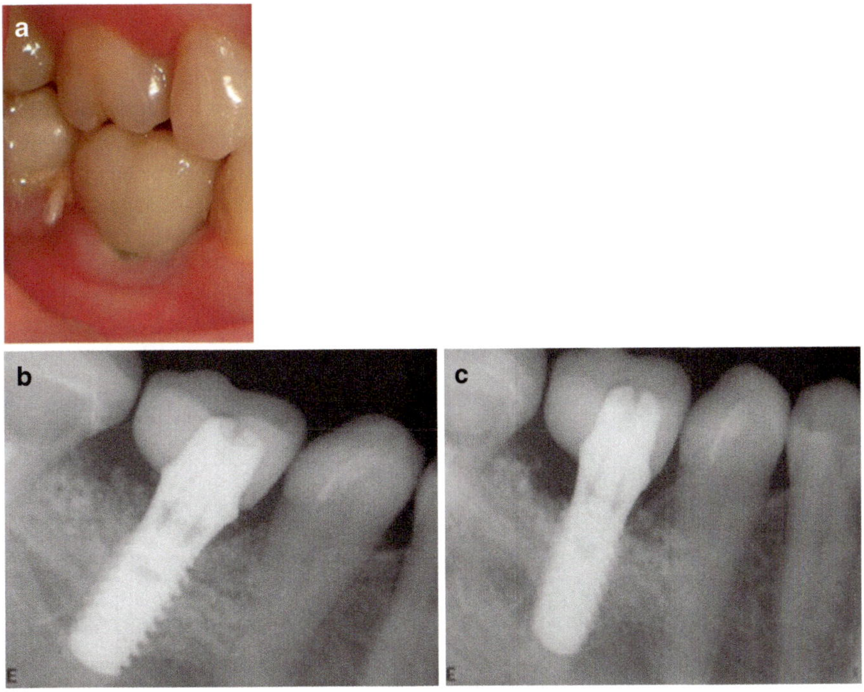

Fig. 8.28 (**a**) Food impaction distal to the implant due to an open contact. (**b**) Bone level on the day of restoration insertion. (**c**) Bone loss on the distal side of the implant resulting from food impaction

resorption that is usually associated with implant surface exposure causing soft tissue problems [6] (Fig. 8.30a,b).

Abutment screw loosening is a frequent complication. Reasons include improper screw torquing according to the manufacturer's instructions, non-passive restorations, improper occlusion, and inaccurate fit between implant components [2]. Screw loosening is associated with biomechanical problems together with micro gaps causing food accumulation that ends up with soft tissue problems [50]. Restoration and abutment micro movement and later on macro movement can also cause mechanical irritation to peri-implant soft tissues with resultant problems (Fig. 8.31).

Connecting implants to natural teeth is a debatable issue. Movement of natural teeth due to the compressibility of the periodontal ligament results in undue stresses transmitted to implants, causing peri-implant bone loss and later on soft tissue problems (Figs. 8.32,8.33). Most of the studies advocate not connecting implants to natural teeth except in very limited conditions when it is absolutely necessary to avoid biomechanical and biological problems [51, 52].

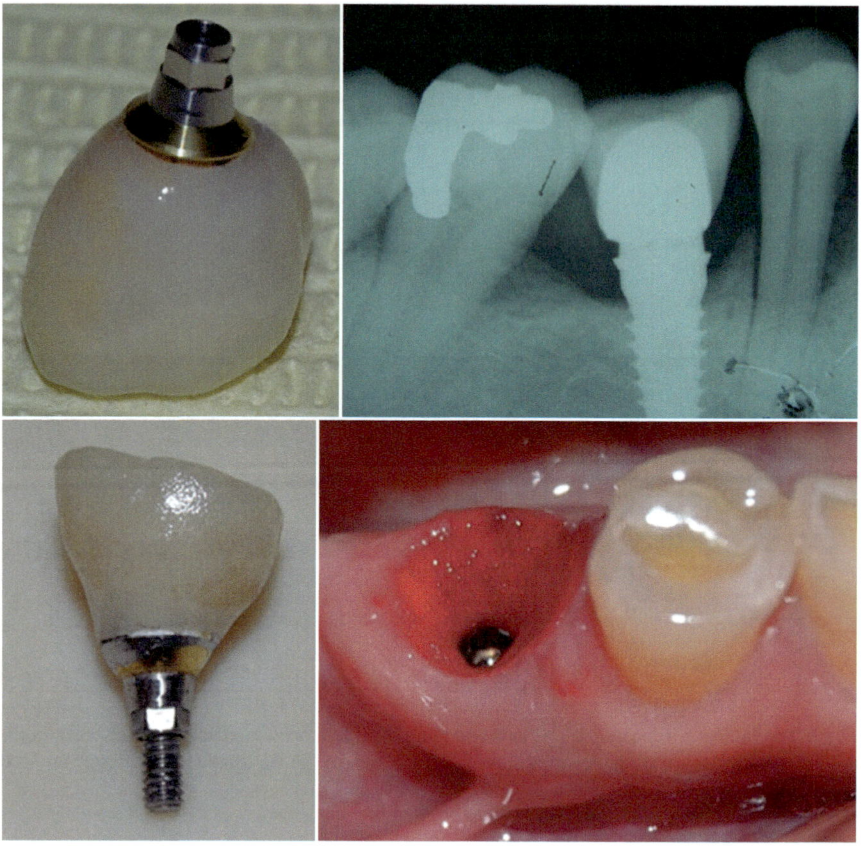

Fig. 8.29 Restorations with an open margin can result in soft tissue problems. Peri-implant mucositis resulting from a restoration with open margins

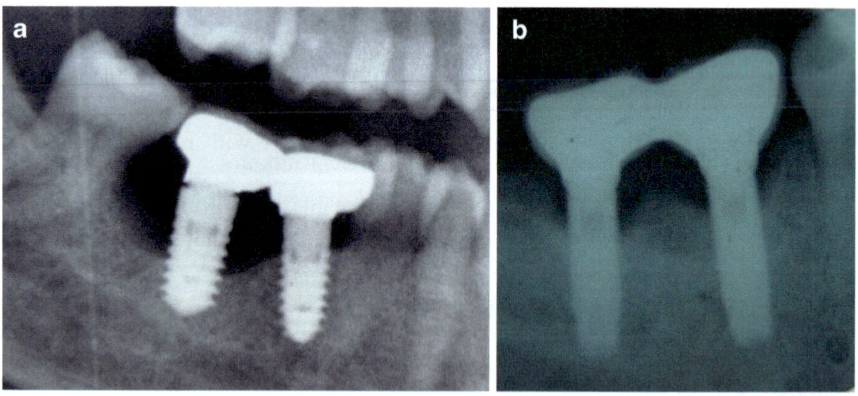

Fig. 8.30 (**a**) Un-passive restoration with an open margin resulting in bone loss associated with the distal implant. (**b**) Improper occlusion resulting in crater-like bone resorption

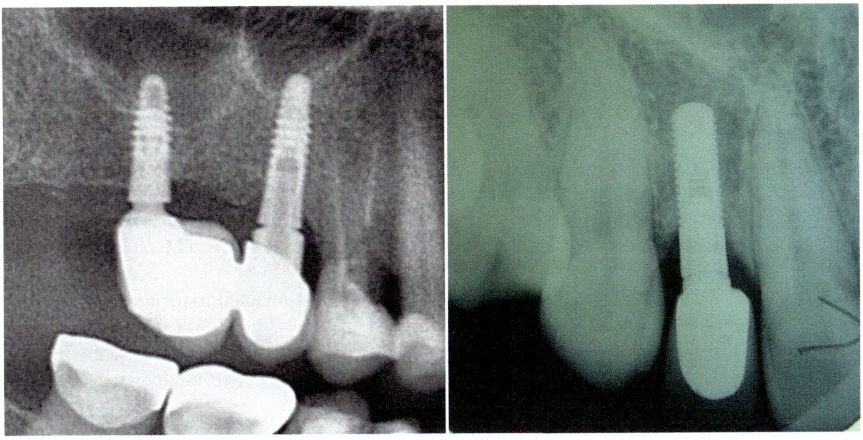

Fig. 8.31 Abutment screw loosening can be detected on an X-ray by the presence of a micro gap between the implant and abutment

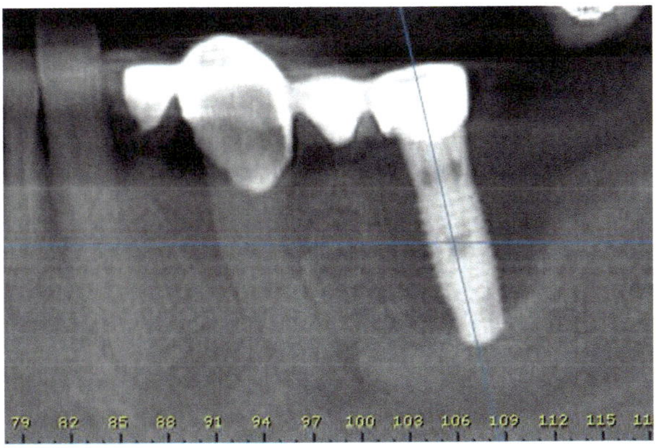

Fig. 8.32 Connecting implants to natural teeth results in bone loss around implants

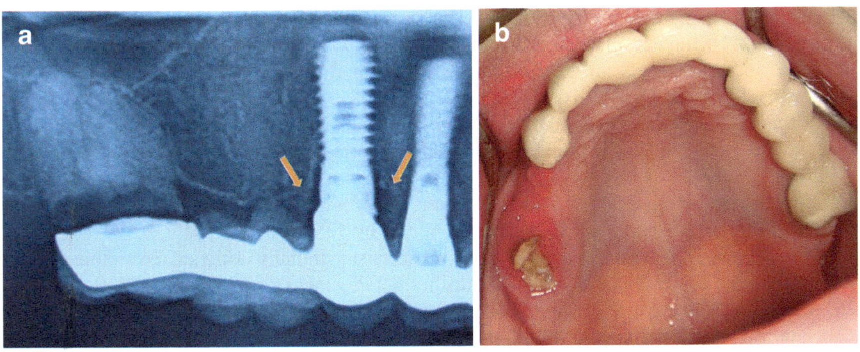

Fig. 8.33 (**a**) Natural tooth caries resulting in a long cantilever on the implants with evident bone loss related mainly to the distal implant. (**b**) Carious tooth totally separated from the bridge

References

1. Khamis MM, Zakaria NH. Effect of screw access channel on fracture resistance of lithium disilicate cement retained implant supported posterior crowns. J Prosthet Dent. 2020;127(4):618–25.
2. Goodacre CJ, Bernal G, Rungcharassaeng K, Kan JYK. Clinical complications with implants and implant prostheses. J Prosthet Dent. 2003;90:121–32.
3. Yazigi C, Kern M, Chaar MS, Libecki W, Elsayed A. The influence of the restorative material on the mechanical behavior of screw-retained hybrid-abutment-crowns. J Mech Behav Biomed Mater. 2020;111:1–6.
4. Chaar MS, Att W, Strub JR. Prosthetic outcome of cement-retained implant-supported fixed dental restorations: a systematic review. J Oral Rehabil. 2011;38:697–711.
5. Kraus RD, Epprecht A, Hammerle CHF, Sailer I, Thoma DS. Cemented vs screw-retained zirconia-based single implant reconstructions: a 3-year prospective randomized controlled clinical trial. Clin Implant Dent Relat Res. 2019;21:578–85.
6. Taylor TD, Agar JR, Vogiatzi T. Implant prosthodontics: current perspective and future directions. Int J Oral Maxillofac Implants. 2000;15:66–75.
7. Bernal G, Okamura M, Munoz CA. The effects of abutment taper, length and cement type on resistance to dislodgement of cement-retained, implant supported restorations. J Prosthodont. 2003;12:111–5.
8. Saber FS, Abolfazli N, Nuroloyuni S, Khodabakhsh S, Bahrami M, Nahidi R, et al. Effect of abutment height on retention of single cement-retained, wide-and narrow-platform implant-supported restorations. J Dent Res Dent Clin Dent Prospects. 2012;6:98–101.
9. Beumer J, Faulkner RF, Shah KC, Wu BM. Fundamentals of implant dentistry. In: Prosthodontic principles, vol. 1. Batavia, IL: Quintessence Publishing; 2022.
10. Lindhe J, Berglundh T, Ericsson I, Liljenberg B, Marinello C. Experimental breakdown of peri-implant and periodontal tissues. A study in the beagle dog. Clin Oral Implants Res. 1992;3(1):9–16. https://doi.org/10.1034/j.1600-0501.1992.030102.x.
11. Ericsson I, Lindhe J. Probing depth at implants and teeth. An experimental study in the dog. J Clin Periodontol. 1993;20(9):623–7. https://doi.org/10.1111/j.1600-051x.1993.tb00706.x.
12. Todescan FF, Pustiglioni FE, Imbronito AV, Albrektsson T, Gioso M. Influence of the microgap in the peri-implant hard and soft tissues: a histomorphometric study in dogs. Int J Oral Maxillofac Implants. 2002;17:467–72.
13. Mishra SK, Chowdhary R, Kumari S. Microleakage at the different implant abutment Interface: a systematic review. J Clin Diagn Res. 2017;11(6):ZE10–5.
14. Rajan M, Gunaseelan R. Fabrication of a cement- and screw-retained implant prosthesis. J Prosthet Dent. 2004;92:578–80.
15. Khalifa AE, Mostafa D, Khamis MM. Influence of screw access channel on all ceramic cement-retained implant supported posterior crowns. Int J Sci Res. 2016;5:2252–8.
16. Hussien AN, Rayyan MM, Sayed NM, Segaan LG, Goodacre CJ, Kattadiyil MT. Effect of screw-access channels on the fracture resistance of 3 types of ceramic implant-supported crowns. J Prosthet Dent. 2016;116:214–20.
17. Rosentritt M, Hahnel S, Engelhardt F, Behr M, Preis V. In vitro performance and fracture resistance of CAD/CAM-fabricated implant supported molar crowns. Clin Oral Investig. 2017;21:1213–9.
18. AlHelal A, Kattadiyil MT, AlBader B, Clark JL. A protocol for screw-retrievable, cement-retained, implant-supported fixed partial dentures. Int J Prosthodont. 2017;30:577–80.
19. Proussaefs P, AlHelal A. The combination prosthesis: a digitally designed retrievable cement- and screw-retained implant-supported prosthesis. J Prosthet Dent. 2018;119:535–9.
20. AlHelal A, Kattadiyil MT, Clark JL, AlBader B. Diagnostic classification and design considerations for implant-supported fixed partial dentures and screw access channel: the ABC/PBC and SAC classifications. Int J Prosthodont. 2017;30:490–5.

21. Small PN, Tarnow DP. Gingival recession around implants: a 1-year longitudinal prospective study. Int J Oral Maxillofac Implants. 2000;15:527–32.
22. Lin WS, Harris BT, Zandinejad A, Martin WC, Morton D. Use of prefabricated titanium abutments and customized anatomic lithium disilicate structures for cement-retained implant restorations in the esthetic zone. J Prosthet Dent. 2014;111(3):181–5. https://doi.org/10.1016/j.prosdent.2013.07.013. Epub 2013 Dec 18.
23. Kohal RJ, Att W, Bachle M, Butz F. Ceramic abutments and ceramic oral implants. An update. Periodontol 2000. 2008;47:224–43.
24. Bajraktarova-Valjakova E, Korunoska-Stevkovska V, Kapusevska B, Gigovski N, Bajraktarova-Misevska C, Grozdanov A. Contemporary dental ceramic materials, a review: chemical composition, physical and mechanical properties, indications for use. Open Access Maced J Med Sci. 2018;6:1742–55.
25. Gracia S, Thompson VP, Ferencz JL, Silva NRFA, Bonfante EA. A new classification system for all-ceramic and ceramic-like restorative materials. Int J Prosthodont. 2015;28:227–35.
26. Kim YS, Ko Y, Kye SB, Yang SM. Human gingival fibroblast (HGF-1) attachment and proliferation on several abutment materials with various colors. Int J Oral Maxillofac Implants. 2014;29:969–75.
27. Ramadan RE, Bahgat MM, Abdelhamid AM, Khamis MM. Registration of maxillomandibular relationship through a fully digital workflow for complete-mouth rehabilitation with screw-retained fixed implant-supported prostheses: a clinical report. J Prosthet Dent. 2023;S0022–3913(22):00760. https://doi.org/10.1016/j.prosdent.2022.11.027.
28. Abrahamsson I, Berglundh T, Glantz PO, Linghe J. The mucosal attachment at different abutments. An experimental study in dogs. J Clin Periodontol. 1998;25:721–7.
29. Nakamura K, Kanno T, Milleding P, Ortengren U. Zirconia as a dental implant abutment material: a systematic review. Int J Prosthodont. 2010;23(4):299–309.
30. Brunot-Gohin C, Duval JL, Azogui EE, Jannetta R, Pezron I, Laurent-Maquin D, Gangloff SC, Egles C. Soft tissue adhesion of polished versus glazed lithium disilicate ceramic for dental applications. Dent Mater. 2013;29(9):e205–12. https://doi.org/10.1016/j.dental.2013.05.004. Epub 2013 Jun 24.
31. van Brakel R, Meijer GJ, Verhoeven JW, Jansen J, de Putter C, Cune MS. Soft tissue response to zirconia and titanium implant abutments: an in vivo within-subject comparison. J Clin Periodontol. 2012;39(10):995–1001. https://doi.org/10.1111/j.1600-051X.2012.01931.x. Epub 2012 Aug 5.
32. Blanco J, Caneiro L, Liñares A, Batalla P, Muñoz F, Ramos I. Peri-implant soft tissue analyses comparing Ti and ZrO2 abutments: an animal study on beagle dogs. Clin Oral Implants Res. 2016;27(10):1221–6. https://doi.org/10.1111/clr.12729. Epub 2015 Nov 19.
33. Papadiochou S, Pissiotis AL. Marginal adaptation and CAD-CAM technology: a systematic review of restorative material and fabrication techniques. J Prosthet Dent. 2018;119(4):545–51. https://doi.org/10.1016/j.prosdent.2017.07.001. Epub 2017 Sep 28.
34. Amin S, Weber HP, Finkelman M, El Rafie K, Kudara Y, Papaspyridakos P. Digital vs. conventional full-arch implant impressions: a comparative study. Clin Oral Implants Res. 2017;28(11):1360–7. https://doi.org/10.1111/clr.12994. Epub 2016 Dec 31.
35. Papaspyridakos P, Vazouras K, Chen YW, Kotina E, Natto Z, Kang K, Chochlidakis K. Digital vs conventional implant impressions: a systematic review and meta-analysis. J Prosthodont. 2020;29(8):660–78. https://doi.org/10.1111/jopr.13211. Epub 2020 Jul 16.
36. Memari Y, Mohajerfar M, Armin A, Kamalian F, Rezayani V, Beyabanaki E. Marginal adaptation of CAD/CAM all-ceramic crowns made by different impression methods: a literature review. J Prosthodont. 2019;28(2):e536–44. https://doi.org/10.1111/jopr.12800. Epub 2018 Apr 20.
37. Khamis MM, Zaki HS, Rudy TE. A comparison of the effect of different occlusal forms in mandibular implant overdentures. J Prosthet Dent. 1998;79:422–9.

38. Ishikawa-Nagai S, Da Silva J, Weber H, Park S. Optical phenomenon of periimplant soft tissue. Part II. Preferred implant neck color to improve soft tissue esthetics. Clin Oral Implants Res. 2007;18:575–80.
39. Abrahamsson I, Berglundh T, Glantz PO, Lindhe J. The mucosal attachment at different abutments: an experimental study in dogs. J Clin Periodontol. 1998;25:721–7.
40. Lim H-P, Lee K-M, Koh Y-I, Park S-W. Allergic contact stomatitis caused by a titanium nitride-coated implant abutment: a clinical report. J Prosthet Dent. 2012;108:209–13.
41. Jung RE, et al. In vitro color changes of soft tissues caused by restorative materials. Int J Periodontics Restorative Dent. 2007;27(3):251–7.
42. Jung RE, et al. The effect of all-ceramic and porcelain-fused-to-metal restorations on marginal peri-implant soft tissue color: a randomized controlled clinical trial. Int J Periodontics Restorative Dent. 2008;28(4):357–65.
43. Tu Z, Zhu Y, Li N, Hu H, Cao L. Applications and advances on surface treatment for titanium and titanium alloy. Surf Tech. 2009;38:76–7.
44. Farrag KM, Khamis MM. Effect of anodized abutment collars on peri-implant soft tissue: a split-mouth clinical study. J Prosthet Dent. 2021;130:59–67.
45. Wang T, Wang L, Lu Q, Fan Z. Changes in the esthetic, physical, and biological properties of a titanium alloy abutment treated by anodic oxidation. J Prosthet Dent. 2019;121:156–65.
46. Charrière R, Lacaille G, Pedeferri MP, Faucheu J, Delafosse D. Characterization of the gonio-apparent character of colored anodized titanium surfaces. Color Res Appl. 2015;40:483–90.
47. Zitzmann NU, Berglundh T. Definition and prevalence of peri-implant diseases. J Clin Periodontol. 2008;35(8 Suppl):286–91. https://doi.org/10.1111/j.1600-051X.2008.01274.x.
48. Roos-Jansåker AM, Lindahl C, Renvert H, Renvert S. Nine- to fourteen-year follow-up of implant treatment. Part II: presence of peri-implant lesions. J Clin Periodontol. 2006;33(4):290–5. https://doi.org/10.1111/j.1600-051X.2006.00906.x.
49. Derks J, Tomasi C. Peri-implant health and disease. A systematic review of current epidemiology. J Clin Periodontol. 2015;42(Suppl 16):S158–71. https://doi.org/10.1111/jcpe.12334.
50. Huang Y, Wang J. Mechanism of and factors associated with the loosening of the implant abutment screw: a review. J Esthet Restor Dent. 2019;31(4):338–45. https://doi.org/10.1111/jerd.12494. Epub 2019 May 31.
51. Misch C, Ismail Y. Finite element stress analysis of tooth-implant fixed partial denture designs. J Prosthet Dent. 1993;2:83–92.
52. Chee W, Jivraj S. Connecting implants to teeth. Br Dent J. 2006;201(10):629.

9 Occlusion and Peri-implant Soft Tissues

Mohamed Hassan

9.1 Effects of Occlusion on Soft Tissues Around Dental Implants

In order to properly apply occlusal concepts, it should not be dealt with only as how teeth come in contact, whether in static or dynamic occlusion; rather, it is recommended to perform occlusal evaluation and analysis and incorporate it into the comprehensive oral evaluation. This evaluation should include both physiologic functions and nonphysiologic functions. Dental occlusion is controlled by the dynamic process of mastication, which is regulated by the elements of the masticatory system.

The occlusal forces applied during teeth contact can either be within the adaptive capacity of the masticatory system or it may exceed the adaptive limit in which case it will cause destruction to the system. The ability of the system to withstand different levels of forces may vary from one individual to another and may also change from time to time on the same person. When the adaptive capacity is less than the applied forces, the resultant injury to the tissues is called trauma from occlusion [1–3].

Traumatic occlusion relates to its destructive effects and not necessarily how teeth occlude. Trauma from occlusion can either be primary or secondary; primary trauma from occlusion is a result of alterations of occlusal forces. When the manifestation of traumatic occlusion results from the reduced ability of the tissues of the masticatory system to resist the forces, it is then considered secondary trauma from occlusion [4].

M. Hassan (✉)
Oral Medicine, Infection & Immunity, Harvard school of dental medicine, Boston, MA, USA
e-mail: mohamed_Hassan@hsdm.harvard.edu

M. Hassan (ed.), *Peri-Implant Soft Tissue Management*,
https://doi.org/10.1007/978-3-031-45516-2_9

Traumatic occlusion can also be either acute or chronic; acute trauma from occlusion is in the case of biting on a hard object, which will result in pain and sensitivity and or tooth movement. Chronic trauma from occlusion is more common to take place gradually and causes more destruction than acute trauma from occlusion. Even though parafunction habits, as an example of chronic trauma from occlusion, are very common and affect a wide range of populations, they are still challenging to diagnose and manage. In this chapter, bruxism will be discussed in more detail as the most common parafunctional activity to give dental practitioners an overview of its effects on the masticatory system, including soft tissues around natural teeth as well as dental implants.

The process of mastication is complex because it combines the elements of the masticatory system, or the teeth, periodontium, temporomandibular joints, and the muscles of mastication. The masticatory system is designed to function properly under the normal physiological limits of forces that occur during functional activities. Functional activities involve movements of the face, talking, yawning, brushing the teeth, shaving, washing the face, turning the head, stooping over, and the effects of swallowing, head position, and body position. The complete oral evaluation must consider the difference in effect between functional activities and parafunctional activities, such as bruxism, clenching, tapping, and nail biting [5]. Based on the studies of functional occlusal forces by Glickman et al., Haddad et al., and Graf and Mehta et al., it has been shown that "the forces of mastication are of minimal duration and intensity and as such are unlikely to cause the type of occlusal breakdown seen in patients" [6]. The amount of force applied by parafunctional activities is as much as four times as those during functional activities [7]. Forces that exceed the physiological limit could be destructive to one or more elements of the masticatory system. This destruction may further lead to complications, such as systemic or intra-oral manifestations, as in the case of parafunctional activities.

Parafunctional activities have been etiological factors in occlusal breakdown. Further understanding is needed regarding the effect that occlusal interferences have on teeth, periodontium, and jaw function. In cases of occlusal disharmony, experiments have detected that maximum intercuspation may harm the periodontal ligament and pulpal tissues of the affected tooth. In addition, this may disrupt smooth jaw function and may cause jaw muscle pain, clicking, and other symptoms of TMD [8]. As the literature widely supports, bruxism and its effects are the most prevalent and destructive dental disorders. Although widespread, even in its late stages, it is often difficult to identify. Studies estimate that bruxism affects as many as 50% of children and 90% of adults [9]. The effects of bruxism are multiple and diverse and may include temporomandibular joint pain and dysfunction [10–16], head and neck pain, tooth wear [13, 17–19], mobility [12, 13], erosion, abrasion, loss of and damage to supporting structures, loss of vertical dimension [20], muscle pain and spasm [13, 14, 19], disturbance of esthetics, behavioral alteration [17], and oral discomfort.

The prevalence of bruxism may also lead to widespread and unspecified effects on the masticatory system. Even though it is known that parafunctional activities are more destructive to the masticatory system than functional movements, it is uncertain on which masticatory system element the excess force will manifest itself. Just as when the human body falls, a limb "breaks" the fall, the initial "break" to the masticatory system serves as the body's adaptive mechanism to the increased occlusal forces. Mehta has reported a concept called the Weak Link Theory, which suggests that "when occlusal forces are of such intensity and duration that they override the body's adaptive capacity, stomatognathic breakdown will occur. If one considers the stomatognathic system as a chain … the weakest link in the chain will 'break' first" [21].

If the break manifests itself on the soft tissues around the implants, it may show some signs of deformities such as recession.

9.1.1 Definition of Occlusion

It is controversial between authors and clinicians in a wide range, some suggesting it is a tooth-related position [22], while others believe it is a muscles-related position [23]. Still, there is another opinion suggesting it is mainly controlled and related to the temporomandibular joint [24, 25]. Maybe it could also be attributed to a combination between all the masticatory system elements' function and physiology. The periodontal ligament has some cells distributed and located throughout the periodontal fibers; these cells are called mechanoreceptors and are connected to the neural connection. Mechanoreceptors have been involved in the jaw reflexes and will affect muscles' functions and how teeth are occluding [26]. When patients become either partially or completely edentulous, the periodontal ligament will disappear after tooth/teeth extraction. With the loss of the periodontal ligament comes the loss of the ligament-impeded mechanoreceptors and their effects on the jaw reflexes and associated muscles. Some studies suggested that even after the teeth loss, some mechanical stimuli still can excite neurons with receptors situated some distance from the periodontium [27]. Dental implants also lack periodontal ligament, and they rather integrate into the bone directly to form bone–implant interface. This type of attachment gives the desired osteointegration to provide stability to the dental implants. Accompanied with proper function and acceptable esthetic results to both patients and dental providers, dental implants can then be considered successful. Failure of dental implants can either take place before loading the implants with the proper restoration in which case it can be related mainly to the surgical phase. Meanwhile, if the implants fail after loading them, then it is reasonable to think that occlusion may play a role in that failure, especially in case overloading exists.

9.1.2 Effects of Traumatic Occlusion on Dental Supporting Tissues

Occlusal trauma can cause different levels of tissue reaction in both natural teeth and implants. Based on the adaptive capacity of the tissues, the excessive forces may cause some damage with different levels to one or more than one of the elements of the periodontium. The periodontal ligament is always under constant remodeling as a response to increased occlusal forces. In most cases, after the elimination of the excessive forces, the ligament is capable of readapting to reverse the damaging effects of the excessive forces. In the absence of inflammation, excessive occlusal forces are unable to manifest significant changes in probing depth, bone loss, and bone–implant contact compared to non-loaded healthy implants in dogs [28]. On the other hand, when implants placed in monkeys had regular plaque control measures, it resulted in the loss of osteointegration, as shown in the histologic changes in rats [29]. In order to understand the mechanism of remodeling, tissue response can be understood as happening in three stages. These stages are injury, repair, and adaptive mechanism [30, 31].

It is important to note that after teeth extraction, regardless of the replacement option, tissue change is expected in the socket in the 12 months after tooth loss. The estimated loss is about 50%, which is about 5–7 mm, about two-thirds of that loss occurs in the first 3 months [32]. These changes happened on both hard and soft tissues and in both vertical and horizontal dimensions [33].

9.1.3 Bruxism and Dental Implants

Placing dental implants in patients exhibiting bruxism manifestations has been mentioned in multiple studies and clinical trials; some authors believe bruxism should be considered as a contraindication for dental implants [34]. However, other studies found that despite the negative effects of bruxism on dental implants, it is still not conclusive that bruxers should not have implants as an option for missing teeth replacement due to the irritability of the studies due to the limited number of subjects [35].

Different complications were documented on dental implants due to occlusal overload as a result of bruxism; these complications, such as fracture of implants, fracture of ceramic or porcelain, screw loosing, or fracture, will lead to implant failure [36]. PDL around natural teeth helps in absorbing and distributing occlusal load produced during tooth contact and masticatory function via the alveolar bone proper [37]. Meffert has indicated that the greater the magnitude of forces applied to dental implants, the greater the difference between the implant and the bone interface. This will lead to fibrous tissue ingrowth to accommodate the difference between the implant and the bone surface [38].

9.1.4 Definition and Physiopathology of Bruxism

Bruxism is a mandibular parafunction that includes forcible clenching, tapping, or grinding of the teeth [39]. Bruxism is a centrally induced phenomenon that is common to all people and unrelated to surface factors [40]. The movement is often rhythmic in nature and may have a physiological or neurological basis. The grinding episodes may be a form of autonomic reflex [41]. Parafunctional behaviors differ from normal functional activities in that they are often unconscious; it is common for patients to deny or be unaware of such habits [7].

Parafunctional activities may occur diurnally or nocturnally. Diurnal bruxism is thought to be a learned behavior, while nocturnal bruxism is considered to be related to stress [42, 43]. More studies focus on nocturnal parafunction because it is suggested that muscular dynamics during sleep exert a greater mechanical load on the temporomandibular joints than do those that occur during diurnal clenching [39, 44]. Forces applied during nocturnal parafunction can exceed four times that of normal function, such as eating and swallowing [45]. Furthermore, the American Sleep Disorders Association (ASDA) [46] suggested that the use of "nocturnal" should be replaced by "sleep" bruxism in order to include the activities that can occur during daytime sleep.

Bruxism has been noted during most stages of sleep, but it occurs predominantly during stage 2 (non-REM) and REM sleep. It rarely occurs during stage 3 and stage 4 sleep. "Bruxing events occur frequently when going from a deeper to lighter stage of sleep, perhaps as an arousal mechanism. Both the frequency and severity of bruxism vary from night to night and appear to be closely associated with emotional and physical stress" [47].

Bruxism affects a wide range of the population. It is estimated to affect 50% of children and as many as 96% of adults, both male and female [9]. Solberg and colleagues estimate the amount of parafunctional activity for two non-patient populations to be 41%, while the signs and symptoms of bruxism in a study population to be between 80–90% [45]. Most adults and children indulge in nocturnal bruxing activities to a varying degree at some point in their lives [48].

While bruxism affects a large percentage of the population, some populations may be more likely to exhibit signs of bruxism. These populations may exhibit risk factors that include certain personality types, gender, and age [49]. Female patients report more clenching, but no sex differences have been noted [46, 50–52]. In addition, the highest prevalence of bruxism is noted for the 20–50-year-old age group [51, 52], and its frequency decreases with age [48, 53]. Patients who exhibit mouth breathing and sleep apnea also may have nocturnal bruxism [47].

9.1.5 Etiology of Bruxism

Many etiological factors have been suggested to cause sleep bruxism, but there are still limited conclusive findings about its etiology. Most identify mental conditions or stress. Nocturnal bruxism is generally believed to be a stress-related sleep disorder [9, 43, 54]. Additional possible causal factors include occlusal disorders, allergies, and sleep positioning [9]. Another speculated cause for nocturnal bruxism is elevated mental and physical alertness [55]. In a cross-sectional study, significant correlations were found between different types of morphologic malocclusion, such as class II and III, and molar relationship, deep bite, over-jet, and tooth wear or grinding. This suggests that malocclusion does not increase the probability of bruxism, and therefore early treatment of occlusion to prevent bruxism is not scientifically justified [56].

Because of its nonspecific pathology, bruxism may be difficult to diagnose [9] and is often measured indirectly through sleep patterns, tooth wear, mobility, and muscle pain. Parafunctional habits have been most frequently assessed by indirect means, such as patient's self-report, questionnaires, reports by bedroom partners, and tooth wear [57].

Because of the insufficient knowledge about the etiology of bruxism, there has been difficulty in diagnosing and managing bruxism. Dentists usually focus on a local cause or treat the damage caused by bruxism. This mismanagement may lead to unnecessary and irreversible dental treatment, with little impact on the incidence of bruxism [58]. As an alternative management to bruxism, some studies are exploring the interaction between nocturnal bruxism and sleep posture. This would assist preventive dentistry by shifting dental treatment from a search for a minimum local dental cause to sleep posture [59].

9.1.6 Management of Bruxism

Management of parafunctional habits is a multifaceted procedure that requires dentists to have a sufficient background and knowledge of their etiology and effects. Successful management must treat both the cause of bruxism and its effects. The etiology of bruxism is often undefined, which makes it difficult to treat. In addition, some of the effects of bruxism cannot be reversed, as in tooth structure loss. However, the underlying cause should be managed to avoid further dental, periodontal, and other masticatory system damage [60].

Because bruxism is widely thought to be a stress-related habit, its treatment often includes stress management. For most people, daily life poses numerous causes of stress, many of which cannot be removed and must be managed. Researchers have supported a range of techniques to manage stress, varying from a personality assessment [61] to exercise [62] to hypnotherapy [63–65]. Other attempts to reduce stress include drug therapy [9, 66], stress reduction therapy [9], physical therapy [9], ice therapy, [67] change in sleep position [9], and antidepressants [68].

While the possible approaches to stress reduction are varied and numerous, hypnotherapy and biofeedback are the most frequent treatment recommendations. Patients who reported bruxing activities were monitored with a portable EMG in order to determine baseline bruxing. After suggestive hypnotherapy, self-reports and post-treatment EMG readings evaluated the results of hypnotherapy. Only self-reporting patients monitored the long-term effects. As a result of the therapy, bruxers showed a significant decrease in EMG activity and reported less facial pain, and their partners reported less bruxing noise immediately following treatment and for a range of 4–36 months [64].

More intensive hypnotherapy and psychological interventions are still in the early stages of experimentation and verification. A 55-year-old male bruxer who had undergone 10 years of craniomandibular treatment and use of a dental split was given a projective hypnoanalytic exploration. The purpose of the hypnosis was to identify and resolve an earlier source of conflict that had become a constant source of mental and muscular tension. The hypnoanalytic exploration was followed by an audio-taped cognitive-behavioral hypnotic intervention and prescribed bedtime practice. Post-therapy psychological, physiological, and self-report measurements corroborated the patient's sense of well-being and ability to sleep without the dental splint [69].

Because bruxism is a largely unconscious behavior, researchers suggest that raising the patients' consciousness about their behavior may help reduce it. Bruxism is usually performed in an unconscious manner, and many bruxers are not aware of their own bruxing [70]. Biofeedback treatment may be used separately or in conjunction with another treatment plan. In a study of three subjects, patients were conditioned to be more aware of their bruxing. The first subject was awakened by a loud tone, which she manually reset. The second subject was given relaxation training and biofeedback. While the relaxation training failed to decrease her bruxing, biofeedback successfully decreased the frequency and duration of bruxing episodes [71].

Although bruxism is widely considered to be a stress-related psychosomatic syndrome, there is no definitive information about its cause [9, 43, 54]. Thompson identifies additional possible causal factors that include occlusal disorders, allergies, and sleep positioning. Another speculated cause for nocturnal bruxism is elevated mental and physical alertness [55].

In addition to identifying the etiology of bruxism, successful bruxism management should include identifying and treating the effects of bruxism. Bruxism may lead to damage of the dental apparatus. This damage may indicate the need for restorative treatment [14, 20, 72], orthodontic treatment [72], and occlusal adjustment [72–75]. The clinician who encounters a patient with severe bruxism activities may consider stress but should also do a comprehensive physical and nonphysical analysis of obvious and unapparent issues that may impact the interactive effects of bruxism.

References

1. Coolidge ED. Truamatic and functional Injuries occurring in the supporting tissues on human teeth. J Am Dent Assoc. 1938;25:243.
2. Gottlieb B. Orban B tissue changes in experimental traumatic occlusion with special reference to age and constitution. J Den Res. 1931;11:505.
3. Bhaskar SN, Orban B. Experimental occlusal trauma. J Periodontal. 1955;26:270.
4. Newman, Takei, Carranza. Caranza's clinical periodontology. 9th ed. Amsterdam: Elsevier; 2011. p. 372.
5. Okeson J. Bell's orofacial pains. 5th ed. Carol Stream: Quintessence Co; 1995. p. 143.
6. Haddad AW, Mehta N, Glickman I, Roeber FW. Effects of occlusal adjustment on tooth contacts during mastication. J Periodontol. 1974;45:714–24.
7. Kaplan AS, Assael LA. temporomandibular disorders: diagnosis and treatment. Philadelphia, PA: W.B Saunders Co; 1993. p. 46.

8. Clark GT, Tsukiyama Y, Baba K, Watanabe T. Sixty-eight years of experimental occlusal interference studies: what have we learned? J Prosthet Dent. 1999;82(6):704–13.
9. Thompson BA, Blount BW, Krumholz TS. Treatment approaches to bruxism. Am Fam Physician. 1994;49(7):1617–22.
10. Egermark-Ericcson I, Carlsson GE, Ingervall B. Prevalence of mandibular dysfunction and orofacial parafunction in 7 and 15-year-old Swedish children. Eur J Orthod. 1981;3:163–72.
11. Reding GR, Rubright WC, Zimmerman SO. Incidence of bruxism. J Dent Restor. 1966;43:1198–204.
12. Gutu R, Spektor M. TMJ dysfunction: etiology, diagnosis, treatment, review of literature. Gen Dent. 1981;29:226–31.
13. Arnold M. Bruxism and occlusion. Dent Clin N Am. 1981;25:395–407.
14. Kydd WL, Daly C. Duration of nocturnal tooth contacts during bruxism. J Prosthodont Dent. 1985;53:717–21.
15. Kopp S. Pain and functional Distrubances of the masticatory system: a review of etiology and principles of treatment. Swed Dent J. 1982;6:49–60.
16. Gage JP. Collagen biosynthesis related to temporomandibular joint clicking in childhood. J Prosthet Dent. 1985;5:714–7.
17. Glars AG, Rao SM. Effects of bruxism: a review of literature. J Prosthet Dent. 1977;38:149–57.
18. Faukner KD. Bruxism: a review of literature, part II. Aust Dent J. 1990;35:355–61.
19. Xhonga FA. Bruxism and its effect on the teeth. J Oral Rehabil. 1977;4:65–7.
20. Nadler SC. The effects of bruxism. J Periodontol. 1966;37:311–8.
21. Metha NR, Forgione AG, Maloney G, Green R. Different effects of nocturnal parafunction on the masticatory system: the weak link theory. J Cranio Pract. 2000;18(4):280–5.
22. Ramfjord S, Ash M. Occlusion. 2nd ed. Philadelphia, PA: W. B. Saunders Company; 1971. p. 67.
23. Jankelson RR. Effect of vertical and horizontal variants on the resting activity of masticatory muscles, vol. 4. Erlangen: Anthology of ICCMO; 1997. p. 69–76.
24. Dawson P. Functional occlusion: from TMJ to smile design, vol. 7. St. Louis, MO: Mosby Elsevier; 2006. p. 49.
25. Pokorny P, Wiens J, Litvak H. Occlusion for fixed prosthodontics: a historical perspective of the gnathological influence. J Prosthet Dent. 2008;99:299–313.
26. Bonte B, Linden RW, Scott BJ, Steenberghe V. Role of mechanoreceptors in evoking reflexes in jaw muscles of the cat. J Physiol. 1993;465:581–94.
27. Dessem D, Iyadurai OD, Taylor A. The role of periodontal receptors in the jaw opening reflex in the cat. J Physiol. 1988;406:315–30.
28. Heitz-Mayfield LJ, Schmid B, Weigel C, et al. Does excessive occlusal load affect osseointegration? An experimental study in the dog. Clin Oral Implants Res. 2004;15(3):259–68.
29. Nagasawa M, Takano R, Maeda T, et al. Observation of the bone surrounding an overloaded implant in a novel rat model. Int J Oral Maxillofac Implants. 2013;28(1):109–16.
30. Caranza FA Jr. Histometric evaluation of periodontal pathology. J Periodontol. 1970;38(38):741.
31. Dotto CA, Carranza FA Jr, Itoiz ME. Effectos mediatos del traumaexperimental en ratas. Rev Asoc Odontol Argrnt. 1966;54:48.
32. Schropp L, Wenzel A, Kostopoulos L, Karring T. Bone healing and soft tissue contour changes following single-tooth extraction: a clinical and radiographic 12-month prospective study. Int J Periodontics Restorative Dent. 2003;23(4):313–23.
33. van derWeijden F, Dell'Acqua F, Slot DE. Alveolar bone dimensional changes of post-extraction sockets in humans: a systematic review. J Clin Periodontol. 2009;36(12):1048–58.
34. Lobbezoo F, Van Der Zaag J, Naeije M. Bruxism: its multiple causes and its effects on dental implants—an updated review. J Oral Rehabil. 2006b;33:293–300.
35. Chrcanovic BR, Albrektsson T, Wennerberg A. Bruxism and dental implants: a meta analysis. Implant Dent. 2015a;24:505–16.
36. Chitumalla R. Assessment of survival rate of dental implants in patients with bruxism: a 5-year retrospective study. Contemp Clin Dent. 2018;9(6):278–82.

37. Lindhe J, Lang NP, Karring T. Clinical periodontology and implant dentistry. Oxford: Blackwell Publishing; 2003. p. 279–95.
38. Meffert RM. Periodontitis and periimplantitis: one and the same? Pract Periodontics Aesthet Dent. 1993;5:79–82.
39. Attanasio R. An overview of bruxism and its management. Dent Clin North Am. 1997;41(2):229–41.
40. Seligman DA, Pullinger AG, Solberg WK. The prevalence of dental attrition and its association with factors of age, gender, occlusion, and TMJ symptomatology. J Dent Res. 1988;67(10):1323–33.
41. Joholm S, Toivo T. Sleep bruxism: pathophysiology, diagnosis, and treatment (masseter muscles, teeth grinding, autonomic reflex). DAI. 1995;57–01C:184.
42. Pertes RA, Gross SG. Temporomandibular disorders and orofacial pain. Carol Stream: Quintessence Publishing Co; 1995. p. 61.
43. Murray CG, Sanson GD. Thegosis: a critical review. Aust Dent J. 1998;43(3):192–8.
44. Minagi S, Akamatsu Y, Matsunaga T, Sato T. Relationship between mandibular position and the coordination of masseter muscle activity during sleep in humans. J Oral Rehab. 1998;25(12):902–7.
45. Kaplan AS, Assael LA. Temporomandibular disorders: diagnosis and treatment. Philadelphia: W.B Saunders Co; 1993. p. 45–6.
46. Friction JR, Dubner R, editors. Advances in pain research and therapy—orofacial pain and temporomandibular disorders, vol. 21. New York: Raven Press; 1995. p. 388.
47. Pertes RA, Gross SG. Temporomandibular disorders and orofacial pain. Carol Stream: Quintessence Publishing Co; 1995. p. 62–3.
48. Attanasio R. Nocturnal bruxism and its clinical management. Dent Clin North Am. 1991;35(1):245–52.
49. Hoff MO. Subjective evaluation of somatic health: coping strategies, mastery, interpersonal trust and ethnic variables as mediators. MAI. 1998;37-01(37):56.
50. Glaros A. Incidence of diurnal and nocturnal bruxism. J Prosthet Dent. 1981;45(5):545–9.
51. Gross AJ, Rivera-Morales WC, Gale EN. A prevalence study of symptoms associated with TM disorders. J Craniomandib Disord. 1988;2:191–5.
52. Goulet JP, Lund JP, Montplaisir J, Lavigne G. Daily clenching, nocturnal bruxism, and stress and their association with TMD symptoms. J Orofac Pain. 1993;7(1):120.
53. Lavigne G, Montplaisir J. Rhythmic leg and jaw movements during sleep: epidemiologic and polysomnographic observations. Am Physiol Soc. 1993;36(8):3.
54. Rugh JD, Harlan J. Nocturnal bruxism and temporomandibular disorders. Adv Neurol. 1988;49:329–41.
55. Major M, Rompre PH, Guitard F, Tenbokum L, O'Connor K, Nielsen T, Lavigne GJ. A controlled daytime challenge of motor performance and Vigilence in sleep Bruxers. J Dent Res. 1999;78(11):1754–62.
56. Vanderas AP, Manetas KJ. Relationship between malocclusion and bruxism in children and adolescents: a review. Pediatr Dent. 1995;17(1):7–12.
57. Okeson J. Bell's orofacial pains. 5th ed. Carol Stream: Quintessence Co; 1995. p. 121.
58. Kleinberg I. Bruxism: Aetiology, clinical signs and symptoms. Aust Prosthodont J. 1994;8:9–17.
59. Colquitt T. The sleep-Wear syndrome. J Prosthet Dent. 1987;57(1):33–41.
60. Leung AK, Robson WL. Bruxism: how to stop tooth grinding and clenching. Postgrad Med. 1991;89(8):167–8.
61. Jorgic-Srdjak K, Ivezic S, Cekic-Arambasin A, Bosnjak A. Bruxism and psychobiological model of personality. Coll Antropol. 1998;22:205.
62. Quinn JH. Mandibular exercises to control bruxism and deviation problems. Cranio. 1995;13:30–4.
63. LaCrosse MB. Understanding change: five-year follow-up of brief hypnotic treatment of chronic bruxism. Am J Clin Hypn. 1994;36(4):276–81.
64. Clarke JH, Reynolds PJ. Suggestive hypnotherapy for nocturnal bruxism: a pilot study. Am J Clin Hypn. 1991;33(4):248–53.

65. Somer E. Hypnotherapy in the treatment of the chronic nocturnal use of a dental splint prescribed for bruxism. Int J Clin Exp Hypn. 1991;39(3):145–54.
66. Tan EK, Jankovic J. Treating severe bruxism with botulinum toxin. J Am Dent Assoc. 2000;131(2):211–6.
67. Blount RL, Drabman RS, Wilson N, Stewart D. Reducing severe diurnal bruxism in two profoundly retarded females. J Appl Behav Anal. 1982;15(4):565–71.
68. Brown ES, Hong SC. Antidepressant-induced bruxism successfully treated with gabapentin. J Am Dent Assoc. 1999;130(10):1467–9.
69. Somer E. Hypnotherapy in the treatment of the chronic nocturnal use of a dental splint prescribed for bruxism. Int J Clin Exp Hyp. 1991;39(3):145–54.
70. Ingerslev H. Parafunctional disturbances of the masticatory system in school children. J Dent Child. 1983;50:445–50.
71. Moss RA, Hammer D, Adams HE, Jenkins JO, Thompson K, Haber J. A more efficient biofeedback procedure fo the treatment of nocturnal bruxism. J Oral Rehabil. 1982;9(2):125–31.
72. Cash RG. Bruxism in children: review of the literature. J Pedod. 1988;12:107–25.
73. Attanasio R. Nocturnal bruxism and its clinical management. Dent Clin N Am. 1991;35:245–52.
74. Ahmad R. Bruxism in children. J Pedod. 1986;10:105.
75. Kardachi B Jr. Jo bailey, MM Ash: a comparison of biofeedback and occlusal adjustment on bruxism. J Periodontol. 1978;49:367–72.

GPSR Compliance

The European Union's (EU) General Product Safety Regulation (GPSR) is a set of rules that requires consumer products to be safe and our obligations to ensure this.

If you have any concerns about our products, you can contact us on ProductSafety@springernature.com

In case Publisher is established outside the EU, the EU authorized representative is:

Springer Nature Customer Service Center GmbH
Europaplatz 3
69115 Heidelberg, Germany

Batch number: 10732044

Printed by Printforce, the Netherlands